YOGA FOR NEXT GENERATION

Orangebooks Publication

1st Floor, Rajhans Arcade, Mall Road, Kohka, Bhilai, Chhattisgarh 490020
Website: **www.orangebooks.in**

© Copyright, 2024, Author

All rights reserved. No part of this book may be reproduced, stored in a retrieval system, or transmitted, in any form by any means, electronic, mechanical, magnetic, optical, chemical, manual, photocopying, recording or otherwise, without the prior written consent of its writer.

First Edition, 2024
ISBN: 978-93-5621-817-8

Yoga *for next Generation*

"Start life in Holistic & Scientific Way"

Gayatri Bhaskar Gupta

OrangeBooks Publication
www.orangebooks.in

Foreword

It is a privilege to be writing this, though I am sure many others would be more worthy of the honour Ms. Gayatri Bhaskar has accorded me.

More than two decades ago I chanced upon a book, Yoga for Every Athlete: Secrets of an Olympic Coach by Aladar Kogler, a five-time US Olympic Fencing coach. It documented how bodily processes, such as heart rate and blood flow, could be influenced by athletes' will.

It was my introduction of how the ancient Indian discipline has found great use in diverse fields, not the least in the world of sports that I have spent a whole lifetime in. Yoga for Next Generation: Start Life in Holistic And Scientific Way introduces me to Yoga for children.

I am aware of the passion and commitment with which Ms. Gayatri Bhaskar has written this book, Yoga for Next Generation, aimed at assisting parents with introducing Yoga to children, she has organised the book in a reader-friendly manner.

Like me, you will find that the simplicity with which she has explained the benefits of Yoga for children and backed them with appropriate visuals makes the book an easy to use guide. Besides explaining the Asanas and

Mudras, the solutions offered for a number of problems will be a great day.

For long, it has been my grouse that only is a very small section of those with vast experience in a particular walk of life is willing to share the knowledge gained and give it the chance to become wisdom.I am grateful and glad that Ms. Gayatri Bhaskar ventured to go beyond personal training and bring this book out.

Here's wishing you productive reading and gainful use of Yoga for Next Generation: Start Life in Holistic And Scientific Way. And here's wishing the book the very best.

July 2, 2024 G Rajaraman

New Delhi Senior Sports Journalist

Preface

It is with great pleasure that I introduce "Yoga for Next Generation," a remarkable book authored by Gayatri Bhaskar. This work is a profound contribution to the field of yoga, specifically tailored for the younger generation. Gayatri Bhaskar has adeptly captured the essence of yoga practices, presenting them in a way that resonates with teenagers, guiding them towards a balanced and holistic lifestyle.

In this comprehensive guide, the author covers the fundamentals of yoga, including Asanas, Pranayama, Sukshma Vyayam, as well as Mudra and Shudhi kriyas. Each of these practices is explained with clarity and depth, making the ancient wisdom of yoga accessible and engaging for teens. This book serves not only as a manual for physical well-being but also as a roadmap for mental and emotional growth.

Gayatri Bhaskar's approach is both systematic and compassionate, ensuring that young readers can easily integrate these practices into their daily lives. The detailed explanations and illustrations provide a solid foundation for understanding and mastering these techniques, fostering a lifelong appreciation for the discipline of yoga.

"Yoga for Next Generation" is an essential read for anyone interested in nurturing the next generation through the transformative power of yoga. It empowers young individuals to harness their inner strength, achieve balance, and cultivate a deeper connection with themselves and the world around them.

May this book inspire and guide many on their journey to health, happiness, and inner peace.

Yogaguru Dr. Mohan Karki
Founder: The Yogaguru Institute
Author: Secrets of Yoga | Food Mantra

Introduction –

Yoga for Next Generation mentions how to prepare your children for yoga. Yoga therapy is explained for common diseases which children are facing these days because of sedentary lifestyle, poor eating habits, poor immunity after covid era, and exposure to blue rays as digital usage is increased, mental and psychological issues and many more. Yog therapy includes suksham vayayam, yogasan, pranayama, mudra, cleansing technique and dhyan. They are well explained with a picture attached to help understand better.

This book is about how to make your child to get into holistic living. Teenage years are the toughest for parents and the child himself. They are neither a child nor an adult during these years and hence they find their friends to be more reliable and faithful to share day to day problems. Over the years, the child gets emotionally disconnected with the family and remains himself secluded.

Holistic living includes everything from yoga, pranayama, dharna, dhyan, aahar-vihaar (dietary habits), hygiene, honesty, loyalty, kindness, compassion etc. It simply means self-care: physically, mentally, socially and spiritually.

This book is a gift 'From a Parent to Parents'. If we start to work on our children's health (physical and mental) in early years of life, it is not just going to help them but to build our society, country and planet a good place to live in.

Index

Chapter-1
Little ones and Yoga - An Endearing Combination 1

Chapter-2
Teens and Yoga – Tough Combination 5

Chapter-3
Prepare your child for yoga 9

Chapter-4
Suksham Vyayam (Subtle Exercises) – Eyes, Ears, Neck and Shoulders, Mouth 12

Chapter-5
Yogasan 21

Chapter-6
Pranayama 63

Chapter-7
Mudra 79

Chapter-8
   Meditation 102

Chapter-9
   Shuddhi Kriya - Cleansing techniques 107

Chapter-10
   Solution to Physical, Mental and Social
   Issues 112

Chapter-11
   FAQ's- Frequently asked Questions....................... 117

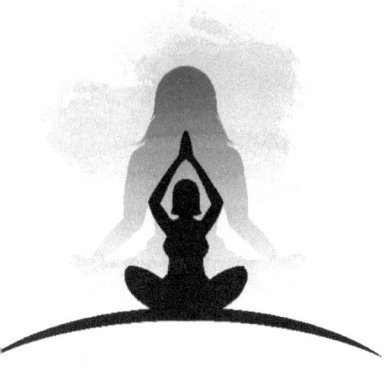

CHAPTER-1

Little ones and Yoga - An Endearing Combination

Sanskar starts as early as would be parents start to plan their family. The couple needs to add some basic elements in their lives like Yam-Niyam which are mentioned in ashtang yog. Yam includes moral code of conduct with some restraints to live in a society (non-violence, truthfulness, non-stealing, continence and non-greed) and Niyam are the behavioural rules for self (purity, contentment, self-discipline, self-study and surrender to the higher self).

Mother and child are inseparable because as soon as a mother conceives her baby, the bond between the two starts right from there. What she thinks, what she eats and how she sleeps affects baby's health. That's why, it is really important for 'to be mother' to eat good food with full of nutrients, rest well and sleep on time, stay happy, control thoughts to only positive thinking. And this is possible when she engages herself in Yoga and mindfulness designed for pregnant women. During pregnancy, a mother must follow garbhsanskar which means giving values to your child in the womb by reading good books like Bhagwat Geeta and Ramayan, listening to soft music, doing meditation, eat right and sleep well that will impact on growth and development of the baby's brain in the womb which will continue even after their birth.

I hear most of the parents of young ones complaining that their child doesn't listen to them at all, doesn't eat well, not interested in studies and so on. My request to all the parents is to change your thought process first. Restrict yourself from the usage of word "No" in your life in general. Process positive approach in your mind. What you think and speak is being manifested unconsciously. Unintentionally, you are not doing any good for your child. Start to give a little positive approach what your child does instead of what he doesn't.

Children of age 3-8 are very close to their parents because they haven't made any friend circle outside and their family is the whole world to them. Doesn't matter how mischievous kids are, they tend to obey rules and restrictions if the mother gets upset and doesn't speak to them for only 2 minutes or if given timeout once.

Whereas, children from 8-12 have started to explore people outside their family and takes much interest to spend time playing with friends. It has its own pros and cons. They may make good friends or bad friends as they don't know much about outside world. Now here comes the role of parent to check who is he talking to or playing with. If he is coming back home at given time or started to take your love for granted. Restrictions are necessary and must be put on kids to make them understand their limitations now and then.

Yoga helps kids to use their energy that helps in the blood flow throughout the body that helps their organs like heart, lungs, brain to function properly. It helps them to concentrate, stay calm, be mindful, have a flexible body, understand the importance of nutritious food, regular sleep cycle etc. Young kids finds yoga really interesting when they are told to become a butterfly, dolphin, cobra, or roar like lion.

Yoga activates and releases happy hormones in the body such as - dopamine, endorphin, serotonin and oxytocin. Dopamine is the rewarding chemical which gets released after completing a task/ goal, helping others, get quality sleep. Endorphin hormone is known as the pain killer and kills anxiety and depression like symptoms. This chemical is released in the body after workouts/ yoga, laughing and spending time with family and friends. Serotonin hormone lifts up the mood by meditating, running, walking in nature, soak in sun etc. Oxytocin releases love hormone like playing with pets at home, sharing feelings with family.

As it is said, mother is the first teacher of the child. I believe a father can do equally well. Giving values (sanskar) to children is the responsibility of both parents. Because if we want our child to become a good human being alongwith successful in life we need to tell them to be yourself, be kind and compassionate to others, help people in need, to be happy for others success as well. It's ok to not get-along with someone. Every person is different and has individualistic qualities. You are unique and so are others. Tell them "No matter what, you will always find us standing beside you". This will help you to gain their trust and confidence.

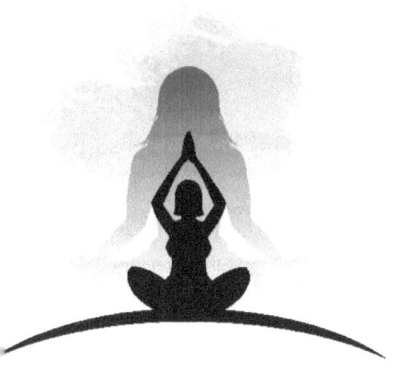

Chapter-2

Teens and Yoga – Tough Combination

Yoga and mindfulness for teens may seem uninteresting to them as they have many other 'important things to do' in their lives. So, how does a parent help his child to perform yogic breathing, asan, meditation and sit for almost one long hour. Teens are complex in nature, they have mood swings every now and then. They don't always handle their emotions well. They are not really expressive with their parents at this age of their life moreover they don't want their own parents to interfere in their matters. Sometimes they are expected to act like an adult and behave in well-defined manner and at the same time they are not allowed to take their own decisions. Yes right, they are not good decision makers but let them share their thoughts when they want to. Every parent think their baby is naive but the reality is they are much smarter than the older generation. They want to explore. They don't want your advice rather look for others opinions, outside family. Visualise your own teen years and then you would realise that just like you, your own children also have a lot more going on beneath the surface than we can see.

Meanwhile, new growth hormones are being produced and released in the body which are causing massive flood of emotions and mood swings. During this time 'Expect the Unexpected' from your boy or girl. Hormones are the chemicals which are produced by glands and get released in the blood stream. Hormonal imbalance occurs when there's too much or too little production of hormones. Several hormonal changes occur in both boys and girls but girls experience major changes in their physical and mental health, not just during adolescence age but during different phases of their lives. Acne, weight gain, hair loss, lack of sleep, breast gain, menstrual cycle etc are major concerns during this time. On the other hand, a teen boy experiences voice change, weight and height gain, facial hair growth like moustache and beard, acne, body odour, pubic hair growth, sexual desire, aggression etc.

Also, a teenager has to go through Social issues like Bullying, Peer pressure, body shaming, drug and alcohol use, parents pressure to build career, sexual activity and social media leads to Depression, anxiety, lack of confidence, loneliness, lack of appetite, lack of sleep, lack of hygiene, which gives us results in emotional imbalances like rebellious, rule breaking nature. And we, as parent blame child for his misbehaviours and lack of involvement in the family. Do not pressurise them for anything YOU want. Though, you may discuss their choices and give them options as you are more experienced specially when it comes to career and relationships. 'Listening' is more important to maintain and upkeep of any relation and here we are talking about teenagers with whom you need to be a good listener, be patient, a good observer. Yes, observe their activities, mood swings, behaviour at home and outside home, if they eat on time, how are they treating their siblings or pets, and you will get to know if something is wrong with them. Children may go through heartbreak, peer pressure, performance pressure which they don't generally share with parents themselves. But their attitude and voice tone will tell you all. Please try to understand them as these are the crucial years of any child which can make him or break him for life. He is going to treat his own children the way he was raised. If one generation understands its next generation, they are not only working for next-gen but building a force of people in generations to come who are physically, mentally and psychologically strong.

Read the mind of your child quietly and try to understand his concerns. Give them a joyful and harmonious environment at home. The values or sanskar, we parents inculcate from the early age always remain with them. Their conscious won't allow them to do anything wrong throughout their lifetime as the values taught are fed in their unconscious mind. After all, home is the first school and parents are the first teachers of their children. With a growing child, parents also go through various stages with them. From the age of 0-8 years, we also become child and play with them all the time. Then from 8-13 years, we become friends with them and start to discuss their friends, school and day to day life. From the age of 0-8 years, we also become child and play with them all the time. Then from 8-13 years, we become friends with them and start to discuss their friends, school and day to day life. From the age 14 onwards, we need to perform our parental duty by becoming vigilant of their activities alongwith maintaining a healthy friend-like relation with them. After practising mindful yoga for a while they will understand that the situation in life remains the same however they have learnt how to handle it calmly. Still let them know - 'You are never alone, no matter what we are always with you'.

By practising Yogasan, pranayama and dhyan, all the above mentioned imbalances can be rectified gradually.

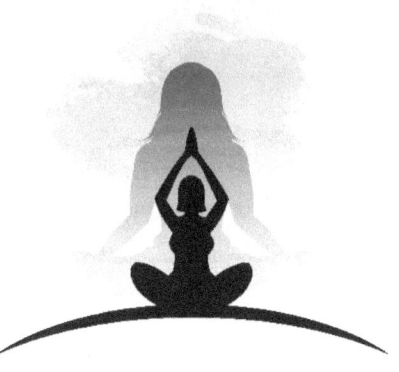

CHAPTER-3

Prepare your child for yoga

Start talking about benefits of yoga in general

Take discussion to next level by sharing the benefits he/she will be getting through yoga. Children are more concerned about their physical appearance than mental and physical health so, talk about the 'glow on the face' (for girls), 'bodily strength' (for boys).

Hire a professional yoga coach who engages, interact and shows his own interest in giving the session.

Traditional yoga may not be their taste as its slow paced and all about breathwork. I would recommend to go for "Vinyasa flow" for this age to start with, which is vigourous and moderate to fast paced. Once they see the changes happening in their body, mind and get the idea of what yoga can do, they themselves will shift towards traditional yoga which is more beneficial for them for the long term. Vinyasa is a flow of asans interlinked with each other with breathwork. There is a smooth transition from one posture to another in a graceful way which looks like slow yoga dance. It works on core muscles, builds strength and flexibility and improves heart health alongwith many more health benefits. You may practice surya namaskar in vinyasa flow i.e, no need to hold the pose, work on breath with each asan (explained in detail in surya namaskar) and move your body with grace. After sometime, many other asans can be added within surya namaskar to make a sequence. Though there's no particular sequence in vinyasa just make sure you start with standing postures then sitting followed by lie down asan. Example - vrikshasan, virbhadrasan 1, trikonasan, utkata konasan, Parvatasan, Cat-Cow pose, balasan and relax for 30 seconds then ushtrasan, gomukhasan, sarvangasan, halasan, savasan and relax. It's a sequence of 12 asan which are explained in this book.

Meditation may be boring for them at early stages as they are not able to control their thoughts and miss their focus and concentration, but once they practice how to do it they will enjoy this gift of yours lifelong. Make them practice "tratak" (mentioned in pranayam) for 2-5 minutes in the beginning.

Don't pressurise them if they don't want to continue. Give them space. Only tell them to do breath work means make both nostrils active. Generally, only one side is active and other is passive. The one from which breath is coming out heavily is called active side. It can be done anytime during the day. How to do it - Place a finger underneath the nose and check from which nostril breath is coming out properly, then close the same nostril and slowly breathe 5 times from the other one to make it active. And now check again if both the nostrils are working properly or not, by placing finger below the nose else repeat it again for 5 times.

Over the time, it will change their mind after realising how it helped them emotionally. Tell them to breathe slow and deep with one nostril at a time and make both nostrils work and can do it before exam, interview, competition, during anxiety, headache or stress. This is really helpful and your child will himself start to incline towards yoga.

Start with healthy diet options. Don't make a fuss of benefits of healthy eating and all. Place all the meal options on the table and let them decide what to eat. You will see significant change in their meal choices after they start taking sessions. Last but not the least –be an icon for them by keeping yourself healthy and fit.

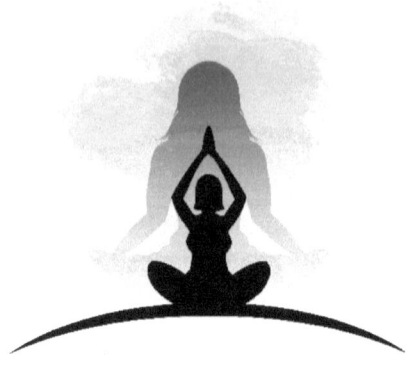

Chapter-4

Suksham Vyayam (Subtle Exercises) – Eyes, Ears, Neck and Shoulders, Mouth

1) **Eyes** – Eyes are the most delicate part of our body. They need proper care from the very beginning of our life. Mentioning down some exercises which will help eye muscles and nerves to be relaxed and hydrated.

Do's:
   i. Limit the watch time of television and phone
   ii. Splash eyes with mouth filled with water in morning and evening
   iii. Read in proper light
   iv. Try to look as far as possible and focus on one point while sitting in balcony/park

Dont's:

i. Do not open eyes immediately and see the light after sleep, meditation, coming out of dark room. Always cover eyes with hands and slowly see the light.

ii. Do not read/ watch phone/play games while lying down

iii. Do not rub eyes hard

iv. Do not use unnecessary medicines if not prescribed by doctor

Exercises – Sit/ Stand straight keeping spine and neck in vertical line. Make sure only eyes are moving.

i. Inhale look up, Exhale look down (7 times) as shown in pic

ii. Inhale look top right corner, Exhale look bottom left corner (7 times) as shown in pic

iii. Inhale look top left corner, Exhale look bottom right corner (7 times)

iv. Inhale look left, Exhale look right (7 times) as shown in pic

v. Inhale look right, Exhale look left (7 times)

vi. Close eyes and rotate eye balls clockwise(5 times) then anticlockwise (5times)

vii. Keep eyes closed. Rub palms together and put them on your eyes in a cup shape (so that there is space between palm and eyes) and start blinking them fast. Slowly open fingers, let the light come in from the fingers and see the light. Remove hands from face.

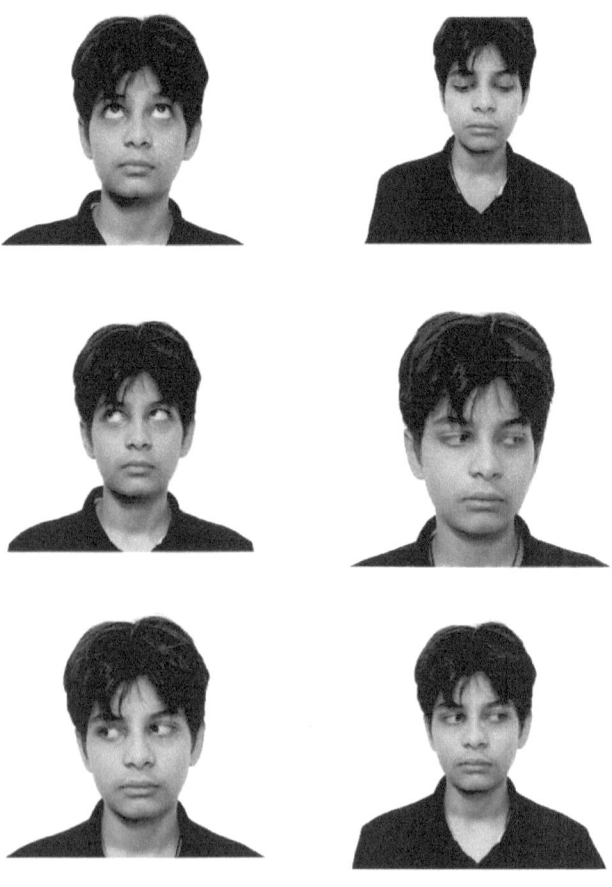

2) **Ears** – Ears are the most neglected part of the body. They have our body acupressure points which when pressed and proper massage alongwith asan, pranayam and mudra really reliefs pain, tinnitus, vertigo like problems.

Do's and dont's –
   i. Do not plug in earplugs/ headphones for long hours specially at high volume
   ii. Do not use cotton swap, bobbypins or any sharp object to clean
   iii. Do not ignore ear pain
   iv. Do clean ears after taking bath with corner of the towel
   v. Try to keep the shower away from the ear

Exercises –
   i. Press and stretch ear at 5 points starting from the earlobe going towards the top of it – 5 times
   ii. Massage ear up and down by keeping thumb and index finger on the back of the ear and rest of three fingers (middle, ring and little finger) on the cheek – 5 times
   iii. Cover the ear with your palm. Now Inhale and while exhaling make a buzzing bee sound – 5 times

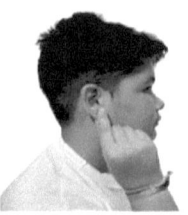
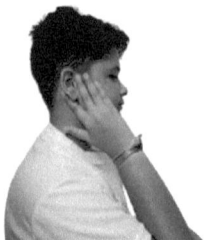

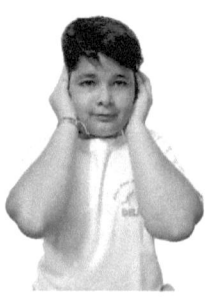

3) **Neck and shoulder exercises –**

For Neck -

   i. Look straight, inhale. Turn head to the right while exhaling. Keep your chin over right shoulder and eyeballs to the corner of the eyes by looking as far as possible. Inhale and look forward. Now turn head to the left while exhaling. Keep your chin over your left shoulder and eyeballs to the corner of the eyes by looking as far as possible. Repeat this exercise 5 times each side.

   ii. Inhale, move head backwards and look up. Exhale, touch chin to neck bone and look down

iii. Neck rotation – Inhale and drop your head on the left shoulder and rotate it towards back and bring it to right shoulder, now exhale and rotate down and bring it back to left shoulder. This a completes one round. Do this 5 times clockwise and 5 times anti-clockwise.

Note* - if you have cervical pain, Do only semi-circle rotation in the back .DO NOT bend your neck forward in rotation.

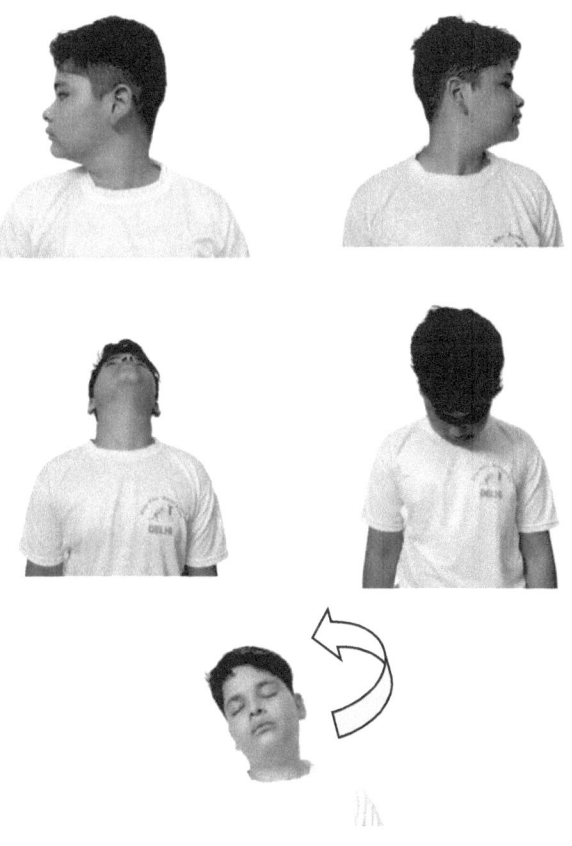

For Shoulders -
  i. Keep hands straight beside your body. Inhale, bring your shoulders up hold your breath and stay for 3-5 seconds and drop them- 5 times
  ii. Rotate shoulders - Inhale take shoulders up, rotate. Exhale bring them back – 5 times
  iii. Rotate arms – Make a fist with thumb in. Inhale, extend arm forward and make a complete circle, come back while exhaling – 5 times each arm.
  iv. Inhale, take your right arm up and fold it on the back of your head and exhale. Now inhale extend left arm and hold the right elbow and press the right arm down while exhaling. Make sure right arm is not putting any pressure on your head. There must be a gap between right arm and head. Feel the pressure on your right shoulder and right bicep. Repeat this with left arm.

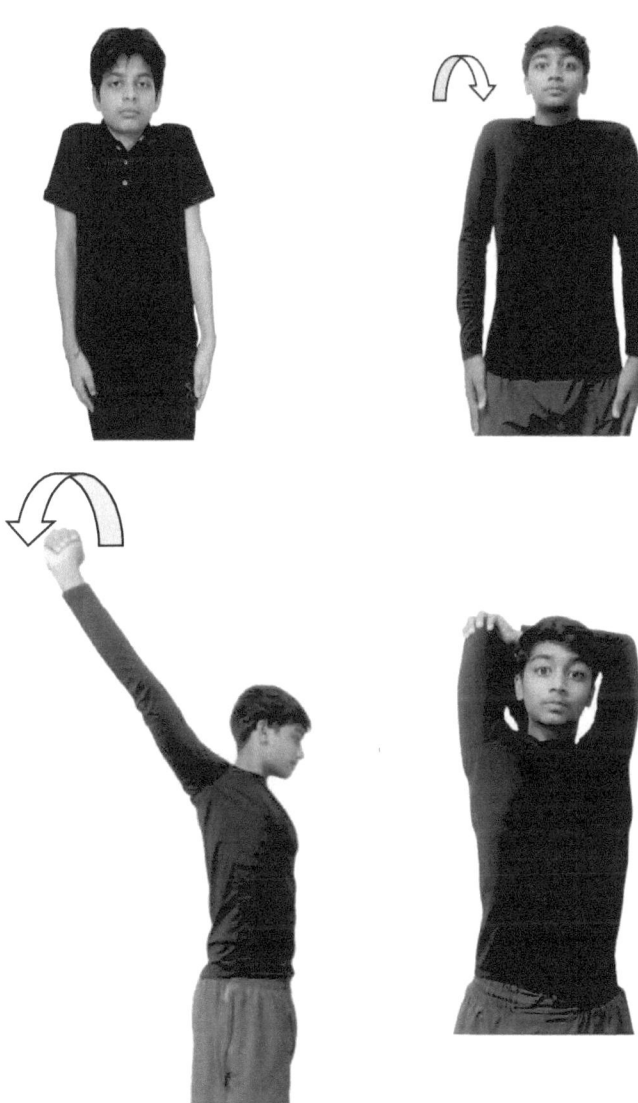

4) **Mouth exercises** – Do these exercises 5 times each

   i. Wide open mouth and close it
   ii. Make a pout and bring it forward and back
   iii. Stretch lips with a big smile and close lips
   iv. Stick tongue out and in
   v. Fill air in the mouth and tightly close it. Move the air from one cheek to other, stop and tap slowly on cheeks. Release air and relax.

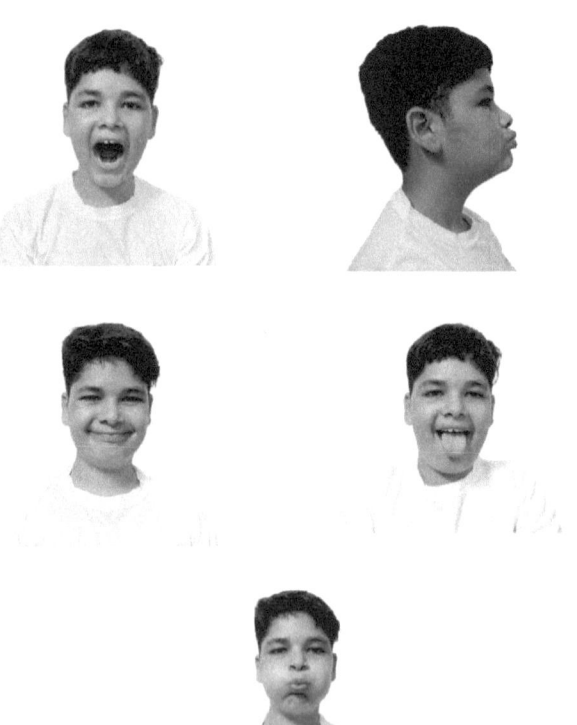

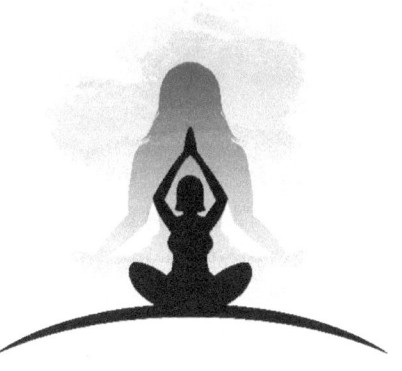

CHAPTER-5

Yogasan

Generally a yoga session is divided into five parts - warm up, asana, pranayama, meditation, cool down. However, it can be customised as per individual needs.

Note* -

The asan mentioned in this book can be performed by a person with normal physique and good mental health. People with chronic illnesses, genetic diseases, or any physical/mental ailment, need to take expert advice and then take yoga therapy sessions under expert supervision.

Yoga is the preventive measure and not the cure of any disease. It removes negative vibes, toxic energies from our body which helps to rejuvenate and re-energise. It helps us to build a strong body and mind with continuous flow of energy channelized through asan, mudra and pranayama.

Warm up -

Always start with warm up exercises to avoid injury. Never underestimate the importance of warm up before any physical activity as it stimulates blood circulation in the body and pumps up blood to the heart which helps oxygen to flow freely in the blood and muscle cells.

One may either follow suksham vayayam (subtle exercises) or can start with - walking on toes and then heels, tadasan, jumping jacks and then Kapalbhati- it's a shudhi kriya and not pranayama as most people think. Kindly refer to cleansing technique chapter.

Note*- A beginner can follow asan from 1-11 for at least a month or until the time body gets flexible enough and gets strength to move to the next level. You may repeat or pratice different asan everyday.

1) **Surya Namaskar (Sun Salutation)** – It consists of 12 poses in which we offer our prayer to Lord Sun with the help of mantra and asan. Surya namaskar is one of the effective methods to combat a lot many diseases.

Benefits -
- Improves flexibility, concentration and focus
- Stimulates blood circulation, nervous system, digestive system, lymphatic system
- Good for weight loss
- Rejuvenates and Energises body cells
- Improves memory and other brain functions by providing ample oxygen to the brain

i. Anjali mudra (prayer pose) – Stand in front of the mat with feet together. Inhale and join your hands together in namaskar mudra in front of the chest.

ii. Ardhchakrasan (backward bending) - Inhale and raise your arms and bend halfway backwards looking up, palms facing each other. Arch your back and spine. Keep eyes open if you feel dizzy and don't overstretch your arms if you experience pain.

iii. Padahastasan/ Uttanasan (standing forward bending) – Exhale and slowly bend halfway forward, keeping spine and neck straight looking forward. Bend down completely with head down and touch the toes with your hands without bending the knees, if possible. Else, you may do Uttanasan in which hands are placed wherever you reach comfortably like thighs, knees or shins.

iv. Ashwa Sanchalanasan (equestrian) - Inhale and put palms on the mat. Take right leg back and bend left leg between both the hands at 90 degree angle from the floor and make sure your knee is not passing your toes. It must always stay behind the toes. Stretch your back and look straight.

v. Chaturanga dandasan (low plank) – Exhale and take your left leg back aligning with right leg. Your hands and toes are taking your body weight. Make sure hands are placed under the shoulders and there is half foot distance between feet. The shoulders, neck, spine and legs must be in a straight line.

vi. Ashtang namaskar (eight limbs down) – Inhale and touch both knees, chest, and chin down. Elbows bend and stays close to the body. Look forward, exhale and hold the breath.

vii. Bhujangasan (cobra) – Inhale completely and raise upper body with shoulders backwards and relaxed, feet flat on the mat. Look forward and breathe normally

viii. Parvatasan (mountain pose) – Exhale, raise upper body and hips upwards, heels flat on the ground (beginners can be on toes), chin touching collar bone and try to look at your navel after exhaling and hold the breath. **Note** *- You can also do adhomukhshvasan (downward facing dog) in which head touches the ground.

ix. Ashwasanchalan asan (equestrian) – Now Inhale and look straight and bring your right leg forward between both the hands at 90 degree angle from the floor and make sure your knee is not passing your toes. It must always stay behind the toes. Stretch your back and look straight. Breathe normally.

x. Padahastasan (standing forward bending) - Inhale and bring left leg forward and put it right beside the right leg between both the hands. Lift up hips, straighten legs. Exhale and hold the toes/ankles by keeping spine stretched, head down and squeeze the abdomen completely.

xi. Ardhchakrasan (backward bending) – Inhale, bend the knees and lift both the hands up and bend backward as much as you can. Now Keep legs straight, knees tight, stretch abdominal muscles, open up the chest and breathe normally.

xii. Anjali mudra (prayer pose) – Exhale and bring both the hands in front of the chest and join them to make anjali mudra.

This is half round of one set i.e, repeat the same steps starting with left leg.

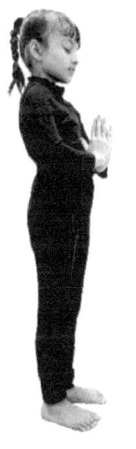
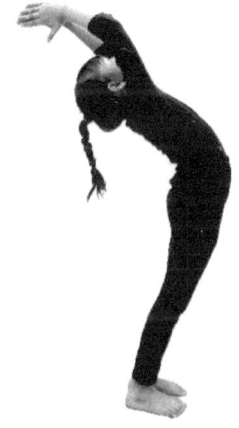

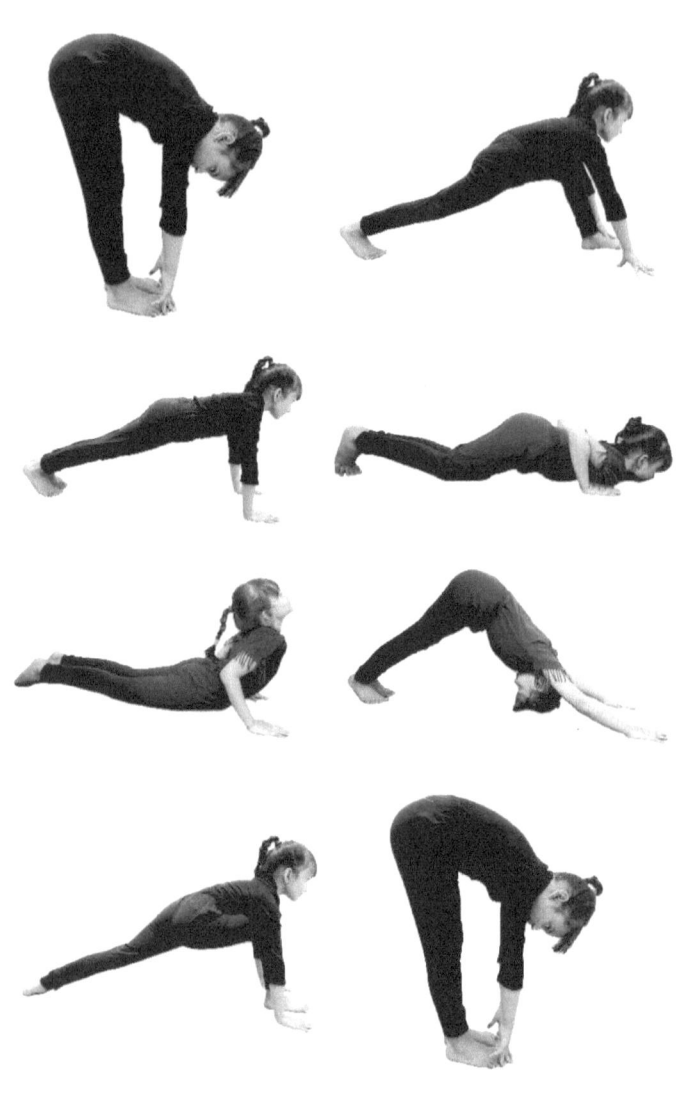

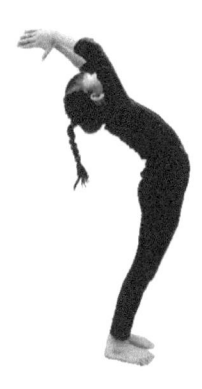 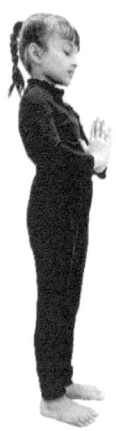

> "Will you believe what compliments I have been getting since morning,'Mam did you visit salon yesterday?" Mam you are glowing, Do you do brisk walking? I am feeling so elated and proud with the compliments" - feedback from Ms Iris Henry after 12 yoga sessions only

Asan done with proper breathing technique makes a lot of difference in the results. It doesn't matter if you are new to yoga and not able to perform asan well. But if you learn the breathing technique, you will be able to do proper asan with ease. As breathing relaxes the muscles and proper blood flow enhances the energy level.

2) **Vajrasan (Diamond pose)** – It is one of the basic meditative pose which helps to heal all the digestive disorders by obstructing the blood flow to the legs and thighs and thus the circulation of blood is more in the stomach and lower pelvic region. It works best if done after the meals for atleast 20 minutes.

Beneficial in- acidity, heartburn, gas, constipation, menstrual cramps, sciatica pain, high Bp, diabetes, belly fat loss

Not recommended in – knee pain, any joint pain, acute lower back pain (slip disc), pregnancy, ulcers and hernia

How to do –

- Sit on the mat with legs straight in the front

- Fold right leg from the right side of your body and place it under the thigh

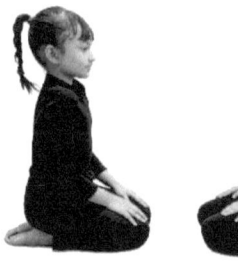

- Fold left leg from the left side and place it under the thigh

- Gently sit on your legs keeping spine and neck straight

- Keep some distance between both the knees, thighs on calves, buttocks on heels and hands are on the knees

- Close your eyes and focus on the breath. It is slow and gentle breathing to relax the mechanism of the body so that energy also concentrates on digestion, assimilation and absorption

- Stay in the position for atleast 10 minutes then increase it to 30 minutes

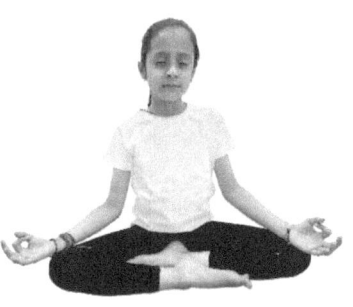

3) **Sukhasan (easy-sitting pose)** – It is the also known as 'easy pose'. Practitioners can sit in this pose to meditate who can't sit in padmasan or vajrasan due to physical issues. It is simply a cross-legged position or simple seated position wherein legs are placed closely in cross-legged position on the mat without overlapping each other.

4) **Padmasan (Lotus Pose)** – This is one of the meditative pose which helps the practitioner to concentrate while meditation.

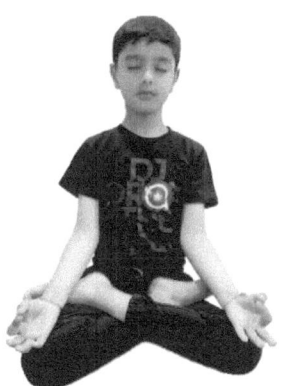

Beneficial in - digestion, strengthens knees and legs, eases childbirth, improves posture, insomnia, menstrual cramps

Not Recommended in – knee or any joint pain, lower back pain

How to do –

- Sit on mat with legs straight in front
- Fold right leg and place it over left thigh

- Fold left leg and place it over right thigh
- Keep spine and neck straight
- Make sure both feet are close to abdomen, if not then hold the toes and bring them close to the belly
- Hands in gyan mudra on knees
- Focus on breath with closed eyes and be aware of the vibrations of energy inside the body

5) **Vrikshasan (Tree Pose)** – It is a standing pose which lengthens entire body balanced on one foot. It needs full concentration to balance the mind and body.

    Beneficial in–Balances and strengthens neuro-muscular coordination, spine flexibility, gives strength to knees, legs, and arms

    Not Recommended in – back, leg, knee, ankle injury, insomnia, migraine, high bp patients keep arms down in namaskar mudra in front of chest rather raising them over head.

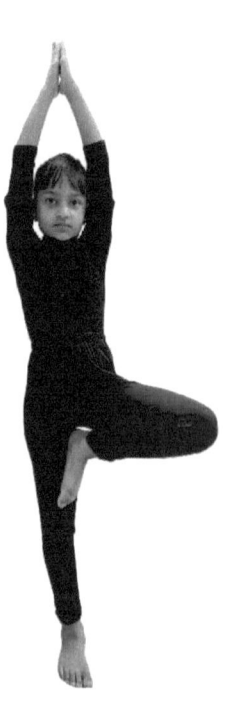

How to do -

- Stand straight with arms on the side
- Bend right leg, hold the ankle and place it on the left inner thigh
- Try to balance by focussing on one point in front of you
- Inhale and Lift arms up from the side and join palms together over the head
- Stretch whole body up as if someone is pulling your hands from above
- Stay at the position as long as you can with normal breathing
- Bring arms back to the side of the body then hold right ankle and place it back on the ground
- Repeat this with left leg

6) **Utkata Konasan (Goddess pose)** – It is a powerful standing hip opener asan. It resembles a wide squat which stretches inner thighs, groin which helps to tone the lower body, also lengthens spine.

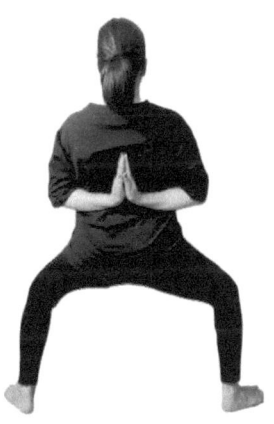

Beneficial in – best pose during labour, sciatica

Not recommended in –

shoulder, spine, hip, knee, ankle injury, high bp, pregnancy (till last trimester)

How to do -

- Stand with legs 2 feet apart
- Keep spine straight, feet and knees turning out, toes facing on the sides
- Exhale and bend low, come to a squat position with thighs parallel to the ground and knees should not pass the toes
- Inhale and join hands in namaskar mudra (in front of chest / over the head / on the back). Stay in the position as long as you can
- Inhale and straighten legs, release arms and narrow down the gap between feet by bringing toes in and heels in
- Stand straight (tadasan)

7) **Virbhadrasan1 (Warrior pose1)** – This asan works on every muscle of the body. It stretches arms, lungs, chest and strengthens legs, thighs and knees.

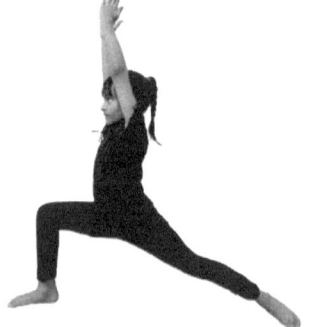

Beneficial in – strengthens arms, shoulder, thighs and abdominal muscles, lengthens spine and good for heart, autism.

Not Recommended in – any injury in arms or legs, high BP, heart problems

How to do –

- Stand straight. Inhale and take right leg forward (nearly one feet away). Make sure both feet are in one straight line. Toes position here are – right toe facing straight forward and left toe facing towards left side

- Inhale and Extend arms at shoulder level to the sides and raise them over the head, palms facing each other

- Exhale, Bend down right knee and stay low keeping spine, neck and arms straight.

- Make sure right thigh is parallel to the floor and left leg stays straight

- Give a good stretch to your spine, arms and abdominal muscles by focussing on one point. Breathe normally

- Stay in the position for 30-60 seconds focussing on the breath

- Inhale, Bring back arms to the body side, straighten right knee, bring right leg back i.e, next to left leg and stand straight

- Repeat with left leg

8) **Katichakarasan (standing spinal twist)** – It is the most beneficial asan for spine and waist twist. It gives flexibility and strength to arms, shoulders, waist and spine. It also helps relieving in constipation by providing continuous twist in abdomen.

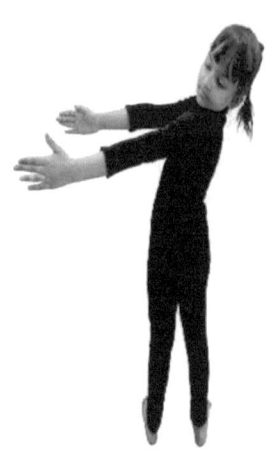

Beneficial in – constipation, back pain, Revives energy, Strengthens spine, fat loss

Not recommended in – hernia, spine injury, ulcers, slip disc, pregnancy, shoulder or arm injury

How to do –

- Stand straight with feet together

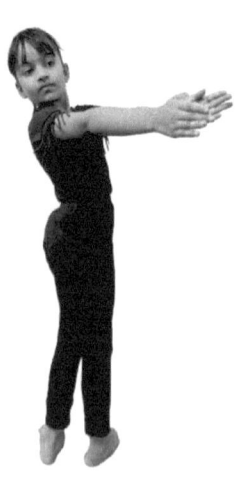

- Inhale and stretch your hands in the front at shoulder width, palms facing each other and arms parallel to the ground

- Exhale and twist your body to the right side taking arms to the back. Make sure feet are intact on the ground, chin looking over the shoulder

- Inhale, bring arms to the centre (try to maintain the distance between both the arms all the time)

- Repeat on the left side
- Practice it for 10 reps each side

9) **Trikonasan (Triangle pose)** – It is beneficial in back pain, reduces stiffness in calf muscles by stretching them, reduces fat from arms and sides of the waist resulting in inch loss.

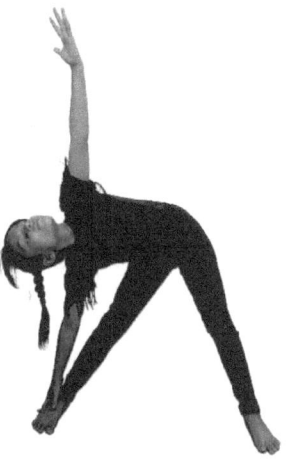

Beneficial in – High BP, blood circulation, digestive issues, inch loss in waist, thighs and hips.

Not recommended in – any injury in abdomen, spine, legs or neck.

How to do –

- Stand straight keeping feet nearly 3 feet apart
- Look forward, inhale and lift arms sideways at shoulder level
- Exhale and slowly bend down onto right side and place the fingers/palm beside the right foot on the ground or touch the right knee if you are a beginner
- Left arm fingers are pointing to the ceiling and are in straight line with the right arm and look up at the left palm
- Hold for 10-30 seconds, breathe normally
- Inhale and slowly come up

- Repeat on the left side

10) **Mandukasan (Frog pose)** – It is the hip opening posture which activates muscles of upper and lower body like shoulders, chest, abdomen, hips and thighs. It also works on shin bone, calf muscles, knees and feet.

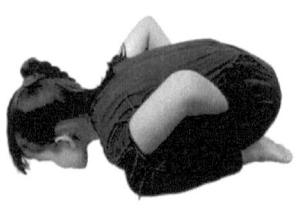

Beneficial in – diabetes, constipation, fat loss in - thighs, belly and hips, tones shoulders and abdominal muscles, increases lungs capacity, good for heart and pancreas.

Not recommended in – ulcers, cardiac problems, any recent surgery, high BP, insomnia, migraine, knee/ ankle pain, pregnancy.

How to do –

- Sit down in vajrasan
- Make a fist with thumb in and place it around the navel so that navel is in between the fists
- Exhale deeply and bend down low while looking forward
- Hold the breath for 10-30 seconds or as long as you can and come up while inhaling

11) **Vipritkarni asan (Legs up wall pose)** - It is the simplest inverted asan which can be done by anyone and get infinite benefits. In this asan, the blood flows

towards the brain and helps calm down the nervous system.

Beneficial in – relief from leg pain, swollen ankles and feet, digestive disorders, headaches, weight loss, anxiety, menopause, PMS, metabolic syndrome, restless leg syndrome, varicose veins

Not recommended in – High BP, heart disease, hernia, neck/back injuries, mensturation, glaucoma.

How to do –

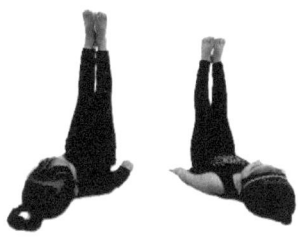

- Place your mat by the wall
- Lie down and move your hips close to the wall
- Inhale and lift legs up the wall (put folded sheet/ blanket beneath your back if you have back pain)
- Stay in the position for 5-10 min and breathe normally
- Fold the legs and move hips backward and put the legs down.
- Stay in the flat lie down position for 30 seconds to normalize the blood flow
- Inhale, take a side turn and sit down

12) **Sarvangasan (Shoulder stand)** – In this inverted asan, whole body is balanced on shoulders and hence entire body will benefit from it. The blood flows freely towards brain, it provides ample amount of

oxygen to neurons to charge and re-energise them which in turn helps body to rejuvenate with new energy. It is also known as 'Queen of asanas' because of it's innumerable benefits.

Beneficial in – relief in leg cramps, cervical pain, good for low BP, heart, thyroid, digestion, strengthens shoulders and neck

Not Recommended in – High BP, heart diseases, acute cervical pain, slip disc, enlarged thyroid, migraine, stomach ulcers, hernia, injury in elbow/neck/shoulder/back/legs, during menstruation, pregnancy

How to do –

- Lie down on your back with hands by your side

- Inhale and bring legs close to hips, knees bent and feet on the floor. Exhale

- Inhale and gently lift both the legs, hips and back vertically up by giving support to your back with both the hands. Exhale

- Move hands on the back towards the shoulder to give proper support until the body weight is on the shoulders. Keep legs straight up. Breathe normally

- Stay in the position for 10-30 seconds or as long as possible

- To come back, fold legs, give hand support to back and bring lower body down slowly and relax

13) **Halasan (Plough pose)** – It is named halasan because the final posture looks like 'hal' or 'plough' (a farming tool). This asan can be performed in continuation with sarvangasan (shoulder stand).

Beneficial in–Thyroid, low bp, heart, digestion, leg pain (calf muscles, thighs, hips), spine, weight loss, strengthens shoulders and neck muscles

Not recommended in - High BP, heart diseases, acute cervical pain, migraine, slip disc, enlarged thyroid, stomach ulcers, hernia, injury in elbow/neck/shoulder/back/legs, during menstruation, pregnancy

How to do –

- Follow the steps of sarvangasan until the legs are up straight.

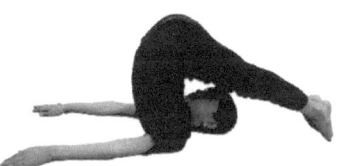

- Exhale and Drop the legs over the head with hands supporting the back. Whole weight is on the shoulder blade

- Extend both the arms either keep them straight or interlock fingers and give a good stretch

- Stay in the position for 10-30 seconds or as long as possible

- To come back, give hand support to the back, bring legs up ,fold them and drop them on the mat and relax

14) **Matsyasan (Fish pose)** – Matsya means 'fish' and the final posture looks like a fish that's why its named as Matsyasan. It's a back bending asan and is considered to be the counter asan of sarvangasan and halasan. It gives relief to the spine and shoulders if done after above mentioned asans.

Beneficial in – Asthma, bronchitis, digestive function, strengthens legs muscles, thighs, hips, shoulders and neck, gives relief in menstruation pain, get rid of double chin, helps skin glow

Not recommended in – Knee pain, stomach ulcers, hernia, migraine, acute cervical pain, heart diseases, high BP

How to do –

- Sit and Fold legs in padmasan (lotus pose) with the help of hands or do sukhasan if you are a beginner

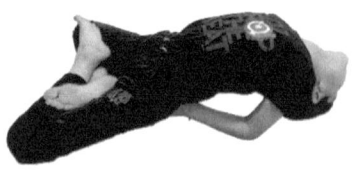

- Inhale and Slowly recline the body backwards with support of hands on the side of the body. Exhale

- Lie flat on the mat and place hands down the hips palms facing downwards

- Inhale and Gently lift upper body as high as you can and touch the floor with the top of the head (crown chakra) by stretching the neck, keeping little body weight on the forearms and some weight on the top of your head. *Advance practitioners can hold the left big toe with right hand and right big toe with left hand making a clasp of index finger, middle finger and a thumb.

- Breathe normally and stay in the position for 10-30 seconds and slowly put head and upper body down, release toes and legs and relax

15) **Ushtrasan (Camel pose)** – Usht means 'Camel' because body resembles to camel in the final posture that's why it is named so. It is a back- bend posture which gives relief to spine, shoulders, neck, strengthens chest, abdomen, thighs, glutes and hamstrings.

Beneficial in – thyroid, asthma, diabetes, digestive disorders, pcos/pcod, heart health, improves lungs capacity, spondylitis, voice disorders, height gain

Not recommended in – high BP, stomach ulcers, hernia, any surgery specially abdominal, spine, legs or heart, back pain, migraine, insomnia

How to do –

- Sit on knees with feet flat on the mat
- Inhale and bend backward

- Bring both arms forward, take them back in rotation and place them as per variations depending upon your flexibility
- Variation 1- place hands on the lower back or,
- Variation 2- place hands on hips or,
- Variation 3 – place hands on thighs or,
- Variation 4 – place hands on calves or,
- Variation 5 – place hands on feet
- The above mentioned variations depend on the individuals flexibility. Number 1 being the easiest and it is recommended for beginners and number 5 is for the advance practitioners.
- Drop the head and stay in the position for 10-30 seconds. Breathe normally
- Inhale and Lift head up, release hands, rotate arms and bring them back, come on your knees and sit in vajrasan and relax

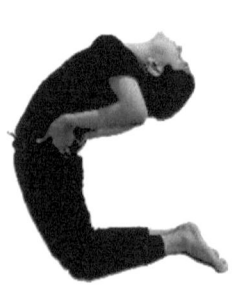 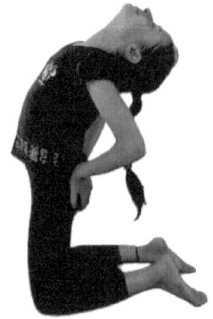

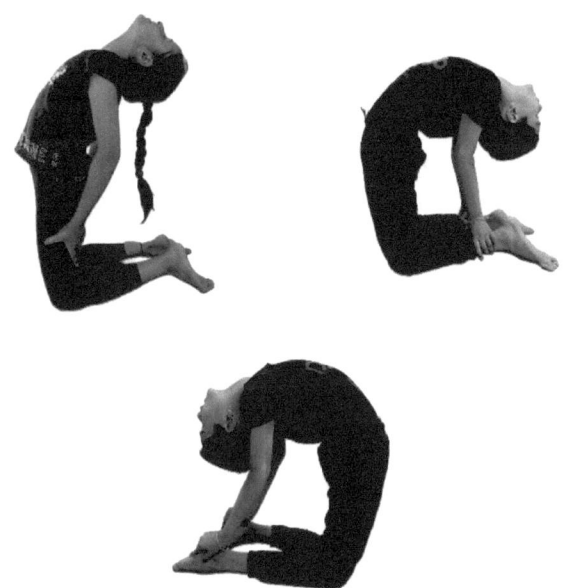

16) **Parvatasan (Mountain pose)/ Adhomukhsvasan (downward facing dog)** – As its name says, parvat (mountain) and asan (pose) is the asan which gives flexibility, stability and bodily strength by lengthening spine, arms and legs. Whole body is completely stretched, increases blood flow to the head and instilling new energy in lungs and hearts as body is upside down. It also helps in bone growth i.e, helps in gaining height

Beneficial in – helps improve posture and spine alignment, digestion, enhances confidence, good for skin and hair, headache, depression, stress, enhances memory, to gain height

Not recommended in – high BP, any injury or surgery, heart problems, pregnancy, old age

How to do –

- Lie down on abdomen
- Lift upper body. Balance the weight on hands and knees. Your hands should be under the shoulders and knees under hips

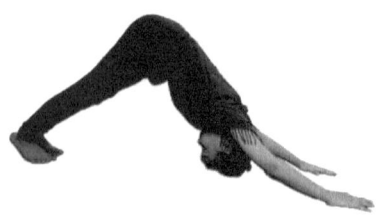

- Exhale and lift knees off the floor and now at this stage, you are on your hands and toes/ feet (depending on your flexibility)
- Inhale and lengthen up spine, arms and legs. Try to touch chin to collar bone and see the navel (for beginner) or
- Try to touch the floor with head (if body flexibility allows you)
- Stay in the position for 10-60 seconds
- To release the posture, knees down and sit on the heels as in vajrasan, bend down and extend the arms straight in the front as in balasan (child's pose) and relax

Note* – Parvat asan (mountain pose) and Adhomukhsvasan (downward facing dog) has a small difference. In final pose, Feet are kept close to each other in parvat asan and wide in adhomukhsvasan.

17) **Shirshasan (Headstand) -** It is called the 'King of asans' because of its infinite benefits. It requires a lot of strength and concentration to perform

shirshasan but its countless aids and cures makes all the efforts worthy. It is an inverted posture so it helps blood flow easily towards head, heart and lungs which stimulates brain to function properly, heart to pump blood easily and lungs to inhale more oxygen. It also keeps the increasing age wrinkles at bay, giving glow to face, shine and strength to hair.

Note* - Kindly practice this asan under expert supervision following all dos and donts.

Beneficial in – enhances memory and brain functions, good for digestion, diabetes and thyroid, good for skin and hair, weight loss, gives relief in stress, anxiety and depression, improves eye sight, makes ears and nose disease free, treats hernia, varicose veins

Not recommended in – high BP, any injury/ surgery, pregnancy, menstruation, children below 7 yrs, heart problems

How to do –

- Place the mat close to the wall and put a thin pillow or cushion touching the wall

- Sit in vajrasan (diamond pose) nearly 2 feet away, facing the wall

- Inhale and interlock fingers and place both forearms on the mat and put top of the head(crown area) on the cushion

- Lift the lower body with head down

and legs straight with feet on the ground

- Do some leg stretches by coming on toes and heels
- Fold and raise right leg and then left leg up against the wall and take support. Make sure someone is present there to assist you.
- Put more weight on the forearms and less on head
- Stay in the position for 10-30 seconds or as long as you want
- To release the posture, fold legs and slowly drop them on the mat and rest in balasan (child's pose) to normalize the blood flow and relax
- Practice with wall support at least for a few days

Note* - Image here shows how to hold the head properly. Beginners may interlock the fingers and advance practitioners can overlap the hands and secure the head.

18) **Gomukhasan (Cow Face pose)** – It is a seated posture in which entire body is stretched. It strengthens upper body, arms, triceps, armpits, shoulders, thighs, legs and elongates spine, opens up lungs and digestive organs.

Beneficial in – Good for Asthma, Bronchitis, lung cancer, frozen shoulder, stiff neck, back pain, lowers High BP, tennis elbow, cervical

Not Recommended in – Piles, Spondylitis, knee/neck injury, low BP, migraine, insomnia.

How to do –

- Sit on the mat keeping legs straight in the front
- Inhale and lift right leg and put it across left thigh and exhale
- Inhale fold left leg and place the feet under right hip
- Inhale and raise right arm forward and take it behind the head
- Exhale and fold left arm on the back so as to hold the right hand fingers and interlock them (for beginners- hold the corner of towel/scarf/handkerchief with both the hands on the back)
- Make sure there's a distance between head and arms. Do Not put pressure on the head
- Focus on your breath and stay for 10-30 seconds and slowly release hands and bring them forward
- Release right leg then left leg and relax

19) **Balasan (Child pose)** – This asan is generally practiced between the flow of asans to help release any tension in muscles, to calm breath and mind. It is mainly done for relaxation as it stretches back, neck, shoulder and spine, gives massage to abdominal muscles and relaxes the pattern of breathing.

Beneficial in – reduces stress, belly fat, strengthens muscles, regulates breathing

Not recommended in – enlarged thyroid, peptic ulcers, hernia, liver and spleen problems, pregnancy, menstruation, any injury in leg/knee/neck, spine, back pain

How to do –

- Sit on knees (vajrasan) and keep palms facing down on thighs
- Take long and deep Inhale then exhale completely and bend down forward so that chest is on your thighs and hands sliding forward on the mat with palms facing down or take hands back from the side of the body, palms facing up
- Close eyes and look down touch head to the mat
- Hold the breath for as long as you can
- Look up with closed eyes and inhale, slide hands back to thighs and raise your body back to starting position
- Inhale and open eyes

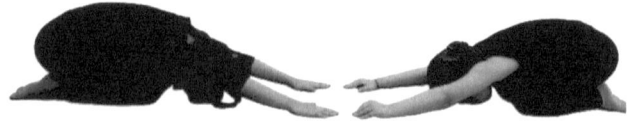

20) **Suptbadhkonasan (reclined butterfly pose)/ Badhkonasan (butterfly pose)** – This pose is done to open hips, groin and restore the energy to get prepared for other asans. It reduces excess fat from inner thighs, abdominal region, hips. It helps in good blood circulation, stimulates pelvic region.

Beneficial in – tones lower body, pcos/pcod, irregular periods, menopause, prostate gland, bladder, kidneys, heart and symptoms of stress and depression

Not recommended in – rheumatoid arthritis, any injury in knee/hips/spine

How to do –

- Sit comfortably on the mat with legs straight

- Join both the foot sole and hold the big toes together with hands and bring them close to your pelvic region i.e, butterfly pose or badhkonasan (as shown in pic)

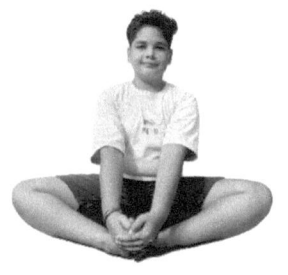

- Inhale and exhale mindfully

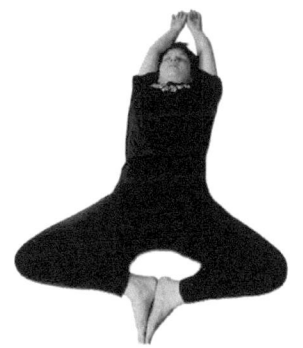

- Now when you feel your legs, thigh, groin are completely stretched, try to lie down flat on the back with the help of forearms

- Spread arms above the head and give a good stretch to you spine or keep both arms beside the body (refer the pics)

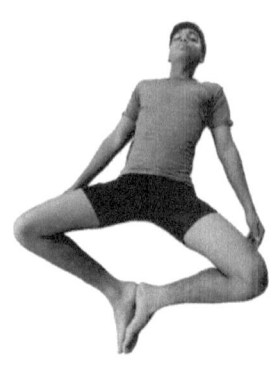

- To release, bring back arms to the side, release legs, take a side turn and sit upright

21) **Marjaryasan-Bitilasan (Cat-Cow pose)** – It's a complete stretch pose which works on the core, pelvic region, shoulders, neck and spine. It is named after cat and cow as the position of the body while inhaling up, takes the shape of a cow and while exhaling down, the shape turns out like a cat.

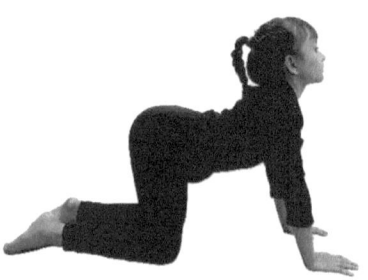

Beneficial in – height gain, loose belly fat, relieves back/neck/shoulder pain, pregnancy, pcos/pcod, menopause, irregular periods

Not recommended in- knee /wrist injury, acute back pain, menstruation, arthritis, piles, abdominal or any surgery

How to do –

- Sit on the mat and come on hands and knees

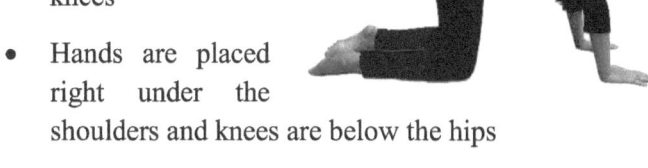

- Hands are placed right under the shoulders and knees are below the hips

- Inhale and curve down spine, expand chest, hips up and head touching the neck, release pelvic muscles while looking up

- Exhale deeply and bring abdomen in and arching spine up, lower your hips and neck down so that chin touches the collar bone and tighten pelvic muscles

- Do this for 5-7 times. Focus on breath to take full advantage of the asan

- To end, inhale and look straight and sit on knees and relax

---

"Thank you Gayatri Mam for your time and efforts you put in the class for a lazy girl like me. I had anxiety, lack of sleep, socially inactive, lethargic and in just one month of yoga sessions with you there's a huge difference in my energy level. Now, I want to go out with my friends, like to spend time with my parents. I feel happy without any reason). I knew yoga is good for health but now I can vouch for it and for your sessions too." - feedback from Sohina,16 yrs old

22) **Simhasan (lion pose)** – When a lion roars, he relieves his anger and shows his strength. Simhasan is a powerful pose to release stress, anger, frustration, anxiety and helps to calm the mind. It stimulates vocal cords which helps in speech clarity, balances thyroid hormones, stimulates tonsils and improves blood circulation around the face and neck which gives a glow and wrinkle free skin. It opens up chest and hence, good for respiratory system too.

Beneficial in – speech disorders, stuttering, anger, bad breath, eyesight, glowy and wrinkle free skin, respiratory diseases like asthma/bronchitis

Not recommended in – High BP, knee/wrist injury

How to do –

- Sit in vajrasan and spread thighs a bit and place palms on the floor between the knees (fingers facing towards you)

- Lean little forward, look at the agya chakra (centre of the eyebrows)

- Inhale and while exhaling roar like a lion or just say 'haaaa' sticking tongue out. Make sure to use vocal cords to the maximum

- Inhale and close mouth and repeat again for 3-5 times

23) **Makarasan (Crocodile pose)** – It's a restorative pose that helps in relieving back and neck pain. It is generally done during the yoga flow to relax nervous system and muscles tension.

Beneficial in – lower back pain, sciatica, hunched neck

Not Recommended in- pregnancy, injury in spine/neck/lower back/elbow

How to do –

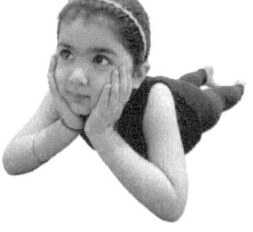

- Lie on abdomen
- Lift head up and Bring arms forward and place chin on the hands
- Continue to breathe in a calm manner
- Focus your sight at one point and stay in the position for 1-2 minutes

24) **Merudandasan (spinal twist)** – Merudand means 'spine'. In this asan, spine is twisted just like water is squeezed from the wet clothes. It gives good massage to the spine and strengthens it.

Beneficial in – back pain, neck pain

Not Recommended in – acute pain in spine and neck, knee pain

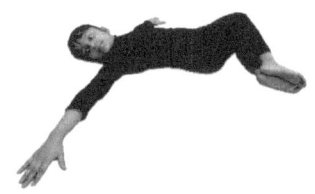

How to do –

- Lie down on the back

- Spread arms to the side at shoulder level
- Inhale, fold legs up, feet touching the floor
- Variation 1- Keep legs close to each other
- Exhale and Drop knees to the right side so that left knee is on the right knee. Look at the left side
- Inhale and bring legs to the centre and drop them towards left side while exhaling. Look at the right side. (make sure to look at the opposite direction of the legs placed)
- Variation 2 – Increase the distance between legs like half feet and repeat the above exercise. In this variation, right knee is touching the left ankle and vice versa

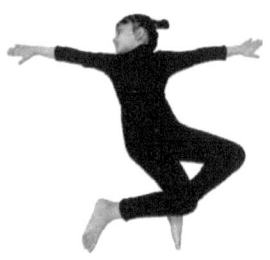

- Variation 3 – Increase the distance between legs a little more like a feet so that both knees and ankle are touching the floor and not each other (not for beginners)

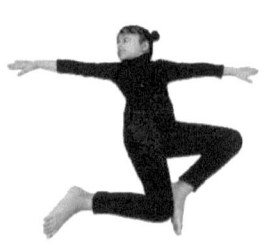

- Do 3 rounds of each variation

25) **Shalabhasan (Locust pose)** – It is one of the best asan to relieve back pain. Spine is lengthened, shoulders, neck, arms, elbows and legs are stretched which boosts blood circulation, stimulates nervous

system. It also opens up chest and abdominal organs which is helpful in breathing and digestive issues.

Beneficial in – tennis elbow, digestive disorders, sciatica (not acute), flatulence, increases positive thinking, relieves neck and shoulder pain, strengthens spine and lower back, helps in irregular periods, bloating, cramps and heavy bleeding

Not Recommended in – High Bp, heart disease, hernia, ulcers, menstruation, pregnancy, chronic asthma, slip disc, acute sciatica

How to do –

- Lie on abdomen
- Beginners - Place hands under the thighs with palms facing upwards
- For advance practitioners - extend arms straight
- Inhale and Press thighs down to lift legs above the ground (you can lift one leg at a time)
- Now lift face and upper body, look straight

- Stay in the position for 10-30 seconds
- Exhale and bring legs down to the mat and come in makarasan (crocodile pose) to rest

26) **Phalakasan (Plank)** – It is a posture which strengthens whole body and tones various muscles from head to toe.

Beneficial in – builds core muscle strength, tennis elbow, alleviates insomnia, depression, migraine, osteoporosis and menopause

Not Recommended in – undergone any surgery, any pain in wrist, shoulder, back or legs

How to do –

- Lie on abdomen
- Inhale and place hands under shoulders, feet little apart, face looking forward
- Lift body up and hold the breath only if you can, else breathe normally. Here, your palms, feet and spine are balancing the whole body weight.
- Stay in the position for 10-30 seconds and come down on knees while exhaling, sit and relax

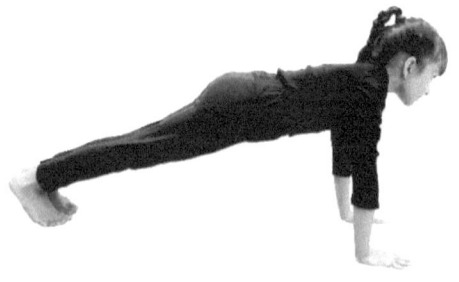

27) **Uttan shishosan (puppy pose)** – This pose resembles a puppy stretching his back. It is a deep backbend posture which releases any tension in the back, spine, shoulders, neck, arms and opens up chest.

Beneficial in – body flexibility, releases stress/tension in back, shoulder and neck, alleviates migraine and insomnia, helps in anxiety and anger issues

Not Recommended in – any injury in arms, shoulders or spine

How to do –
- Lie down on abdomen
- Inhale and Lift up body and come on knees and palms. Make sure Knees are under the hips and palms under shoulders with fingers wide open
- Exhale and move hips backward towards heels
- Press down forearms to the mat
- Touch chin and chest down. Stretch spine and bring arms forward and hips up. Keep knees under hips and feet flat on the ground and look forward
- Stretch and lengthen the spine as much as you can
- Stay in the position for 10-30 seconds
- To release, stretch arms forward, bring your body down on the mat and relax

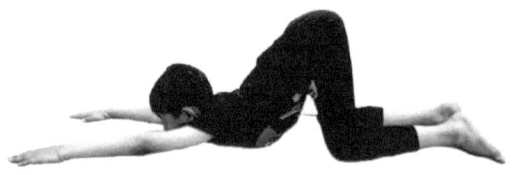

28) **Chakrasan (Wheel pose)** – In this backbending pose, whole body looks like a wheel and that's how its named. It is a complete asan to open up chest, heart, lungs, abdominal muscles. It stretches arms and legs giving a nice curvature to the spine.

Beneficial in – gaining height, cold and flu, anger and stress relief, digestive disorders, fat loss

Not Recommended in – high/low BP, back/spine/wrist injury, hernia, heart issues, pregnancy, migraine

How to do –

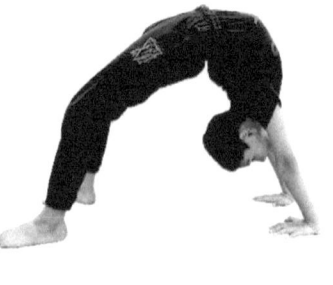

- Lie down on your back
- Inhale, fold up legs so that feet are flat on the floor and close to hips
- Exhale, place hands close to the ears so that fingers are pointing towards your shoulder. Note- Beginners can wrap the hands around the head and interlock fingers

- Inhale, lift upper body (chest) above the floor and place top of the head on the mat (Beginners interlocked hands covers the head)
- Exhale and come down, Repeat to lift upper body for about 5-7 times initially to gain the strength in spine and arms (Beginners- Do this for few days)
- When you feel comfortable, press down hands and feet onto the mat, inhale and lift upper body, abdomen, pelvic region and thighs. Make sure the body weight is balanced more on hands.
- Let your head hang in a stable position. Do not strain your neck.
- To release the pose, drop down head first and then rest of the body slowly and gently.

29) **Ardh-pinch Mayurasan (Dolphin pose)** – This pose is very much similar to downward dog pose except that instead of hands, forearms are on the floor which looks like a dolphin jumping in the sea. This pose helps in lengthening of spine and neck which helps in relieving the pain. It also helps in providing good blood circulation to the brain which activates the nervous system and neurons.

Beneficial in – strengthens spine, arms, shoulders and legs, activates nervous system, circulatory system and cardiac system, reliefs anger issues

Not Recommended in – any injury in spine/arms/neck, high/low BP, heart issues

How to do –

- Lie down on abdomen

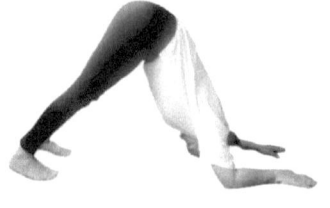

- Place hands under the shoulders with wide open fingers and come on toes

- Inhale and put pressure on hands and lift body up as in plank pose

- Variation 1- Keep both the feet grounded. Place forearms down flat on the mat and touch the head to the mat (refer pic1)

- Variation 2 - Stay on toes, place forearms on the mat, make a fist of both hands. Here, head isn't touching the mat. hold the pose(refer pic 2)

- Hold breath after exhalation.

- Beginners can breathe normally while looking at the navel

- To release- sit on the knees, close eyes and relax

30) **Savasan (Corpse pose)** - It is a relaxing posture, performed at the end of the session which acts as a cool down after yogasan and pranayam. It prepares you for meditation for complete relaxation. As it's name says, 'Sava' means 'dead', the body lies down on the back, legs straight, arms on the sides, all muscles are loosened up in a relaxed manner, it

looks like a corpse. And here, one has to let go of all the fears, anxieties, worries by surrendering self to the higher power. After asana, the energy flow in the body is too high and pranayam chanelizes the flow of energy and then meditation helps to settle down this energy in the body bringing peace and calmness to body, mind and soul by re-energising immune system. This pose looks easy but it's not. It's really hard for beginners to stay immobile for 10 minutes and stay focused on the breath and energy flow.

Beneficial in - boosting immune system, nervous system, reducing blood pressure, increases energy level and focus, reduces fatigue, insomnia, anger issues.

Not Recommended in – severe respiratory conditions, shoulder/neck/back/hips/legs pain.

How to do -

1) Lie down on the mat with your back straight.

2) Stretch your legs and keep them half feet apart

3) Keep arms beside your body with palms facing upwards

4) Eyes closed and Neck and shoulders relaxed

5) Breathe slowly and release all the tension from the body. There shouldn't be any stiffness remain in any part of the body

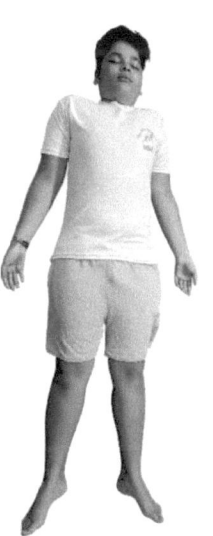

6) Keep your focus on the meditative voice/sound/music or follow the directions of your instructor or

7) If you are self -practising, then focus on inhalation and exhalation and de stress body and mind

8) Stay in the position for 5-10 minutes

9) Come back to conscious and move your fingers

10) Turn right side and sit down with eyes remain closed

11) Rub your palms together and place them on the face, feel the energy and slowly open your eyes and see the light from within the fingers

12) Join hands in namaskar pose. Pay Gratitude to the Universe for showing us spiritual path, for every breath we take and for everything we are blessed with. Now be thankful to the Mother Earth for feeding and nourishing us.

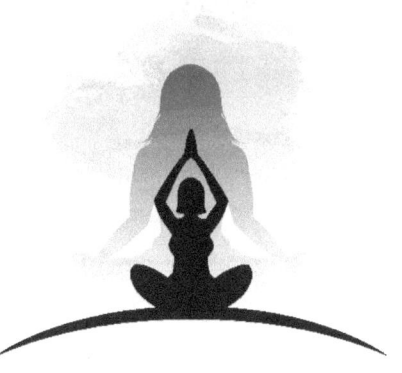

Chapter-6

Pranayama

Pranayama is a rhythmic breathing exercise done with full concentration. It has innumerable benefits if done properly. Slow and rhythmic breathing can be done anytime during the day. Since we all breathe 24 hrs a day, it's a continuous process and one cannot live without it. There's no harm in focussing on breath to get its maximum benefit anytime you want. But, if you want to do proper pranayama, you need to follow its rules and timings. Notice your breath right now by keeping index finger just below the nose. Which nostril is working? Left or Right? Are you taking enough oxygen and giving out full carbon-dioxide? And I am sure the answer is No, because in our daily routine we don't really focus on our breath and hence the breathing pattern is shallow. Which is why it's important for us to include yoga and pranayama in our daily routine.

Pranayama means 'breath control' and breath is called prana energy. Our ancient books have mentioned many pranayam in which we learn how to control prana while inhalation, exhalation, and hold the energy inside and outside the body. It has to be practised under expert supervision.

I have seen many people getting benefitted by different breathing techniques. One of my student was always perplexed and lost. While doing asan also, her mind was distorted, which I could easily see. So I changed my class pattern for few days. We started the class with 30 minutes pranayam and 45 minutes of meditation only and no asan. After some days she was able to focus and concentrate better. It helped her to de-clutter her mind from various distractions. Her restless mind is more calm and composed. She started to feel new energy within. And then she was able to do asan along with proper breathing and got the desired results.

> "Thank you Gayatri Mam I liked the way you designed the class as per my needs. Your sessions are really helpful as they gave me the opportunity to learn mindfulness and different ways to meditate. I appreciate being able to speak openly and honestly and discuss my issues which has been causing me stress and anxiety. I found you really easy to talk to and will continue to make time to meditate as I feel that has made me a lot calmer and helped me with my learning pressure "- feedback from Ms. Sumitra, UPSC aspirant

1) **Bhastrika (Bellow Breath)** – It is a powerful yogic breathing which generates heat and energy in the body by providing ample oxygen to the cells and take out carbon dioxide and other toxins from the

blood which helps in healing, rejuvenating and activation of the cells.

Note* - By inhaling and exhaling rapidly, one may feel dizzy in the beginning, stop the practice immediately and start to breathe normally with eyes open. You may start again after taking a short break of 2 minutes or so. Start with only 20 breaths in one go and gradually increase it.

Beneficial in – Chronic fatique syndrome (CFS), asthma, blood disorders, thyroid, stammering/stuttering, improves eye sight

Not Recommended in – high BP, extreme summers, stress/anxiety, abdominal pain, pregnancy, menstruation, hernia, ulcer, heart issues, vertigo, glaucoma, epilepsy, any recent abdominal surgery

How to do –

- Sit comfortably in sukhasan, vajrasan or padmasan

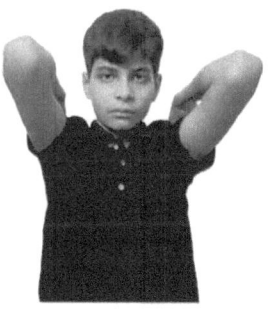

- Close eyes and focus on breath for 1 minute

- Open eyes, inhale and take arms up and bring them down with fast exhalation

- Forcefully but gently inhale and exhale (keep a tissue with you as you might need it here). Abdomen fills up with oxygen and it expands when you inhale and it contracts when you exhale and takes out the toxins from the body

- Practice this for 20 breaths initially then gradually increase it. To maintain the rhythm, keep the focus on the breath

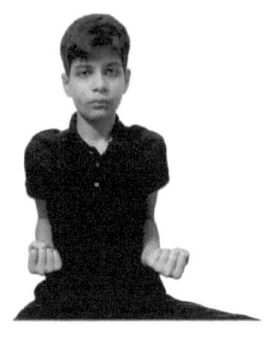

- Make sure you don't overdo it specially during summers as it produces heat in the body

2) **Samvritti Pranayam (Rhythmic breathing)** – It is a slow breathing practice in which breath from right and left nostril is activated and focus shifts to inhalation, hold and exhalation which is happening for equal duration or rhythmically. Slow breathing enhances the pran flow (oxygen) in the body, reaches to every part/organ/cell of the body which helps to reduce stress and anxiety symptoms anywhere and anytime.

  ✓ A quick tip –
  - Do this pranayama before exam, interview or any important meeting, you will feel confident and increased memory power

Beneficial in – BP, diabetes, Thyroid, calms mind, energizes body, self-awareness, pre-preparation for meditation

Not Recommended in – High Bp(do not hold breath), pregnant women (don't inhale and exhale deep/for longer period), depression

How to do –

- Sit in comfortable position on the mat or chair, keeping spine and neck straight
- Close eyes and start to breathe normally. Hands in gyan mudra on the knees
- When you are ready, take a slow and deep inhalation and start counting in mind 1…2…3…4, make sure to count in rhythm
- Now, hold the breath and count for 4 again in the same pattern
- Exhale slowly and count for 4 (in mind) and keep the focus on counting the breath
- Hold the breath for 4 counts
- Repeat - inhale, hold, exhale, hold for 4 counts in equal duration for about 10 times

3) **Deergh pranayama (Deep Breathing)** – It simply means 'long breathing'. It is good practice for beginners to channelize the flow of prana in the body. With slow and proper breathing, oxygen reaches to every organ and every part of the body which helps in many ways like – de-stress body and mind, rejuvenate cells, harmonizes the energy flow only if done mindfully. When you breathe with full awareness, you help your body to get enough oxygen which is the food for our body cells. Hence, the

rejuvenated cells helps to kill all the toxins and gives new energy to you.

Beneficial in - High BP, body pains, relaxes nervous system, insomnia, improves immune system, constipation, indigestion, cold and flu

Not Recommended in – respiratory problems (consult doctor and then do it under supervision)

How to do –

- Sit in comfortable position – vajrasan, sukhasan or padmasan
- Keep spine and neck straight, hands in gyan mudra on knees
- Close eyes and focus on normal breathing pattern
- Inhale slowly through nose, let the oxygen flow down to throat, chest, lungs and belly. Let your belly be filled with ample amount of oxygen and let it expand as much as possible
- Keep complete focus on breath
- Now exhale slowly starting from belly, lungs, chest, throat and nose
- Try to squeeze the belly button back to the spine while exhaling
- Repeat this for 20 times in the beginning

4) **Suryabhedna (Right nostril breathing)** - This pranayama activates surya nadi or right nostril which produces heat in the body. As its name says, surya

means 'Sun' which is the symbol of heat energy. This pranayama is helpful in getting rid of all impurities/toxins from the body.

Beneficial in – cold and flu, sinus, low BP, indigestion, boosts immunity

Not Recommended in - extreme summer, fever, high BP

How to do –

- Sit in comfortable position- vajrasan, sukhasan or padmasan
- Hands on knee in gyan mudra
- Close eyes and focus on breath for 2 minutes
- Close the left nostril with first two fingers of right hand (index and middle finger)
- Start inhaling and exhaling from right nostril only
- Take slow and deep breathing
- Practice this for 3-5 minutes and relax

5) **Anulom vilom/ Nadishodhan (Alternate Breathing)** – It is the yogic breathing practice in which inhalation and exhalation is done alternatively from each nostril. With this breathing technique, both nadis- surya-chandra or ida-pingala or right-left nostril gets activated and there is a free flow of prana in the energy channel which is called sushumna nadi or the spine.

Beneficial in – Chronic fatigue syndrome (CFS), boosts immune system, nervous system, releases stress, anxiety and depression

Not Recommended in – acute asthma, high BP(under supervision), ulcers, hernia, abdominal pain, during pregnancy (don't hold breath)

How to do –

- Sit in comfortable position- vajrasan, sukhasan or padmasan

- Close eyes and focus on breath

- Keep left or right hand (which is not dominating) on knee in gyan mudra

- Make Vishnu mudra with the other hand by folding index and middle fingers inwards touching the base of the thumb

- Close your right nostril with thumb and breathe out completely through left nostril

- Inhale for 4 counts from left nostril

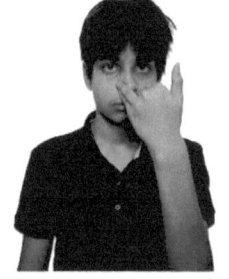

- Close left nostril with ring finger and little finger so that both nostrils are now closed and hold the breath for count of 8

- Keeping left nostril closed, release right nostril and exhale completely for count of 4
- With your left nostril closed, inhale through your right to a count of 4
- Close both nostrils and hold your breath for a count of 8
- Keeping your right nostril closed, release your fingers from your left nostril and breathe out completely for a count of 4.
- This completes round one i.e, left inhale-hold-right exhale-right inhale-hold-left exhale (4-8-4-4-8-4). Hold breath double the time you inhale and exhale. Continue this exercise for 3-10 minutes

Note* –

i. Beginners can do count of 4 instead of 8 while holding breath

ii. In winters, start by closing left nostril and inhale from right

6) **Bhramri (Buzzing bee)** - In this pranayama, buzzing bee sound is produced while exhaling. It has innumerable benefits such as when the vibrations of this sound echoes inside the body with eyes, ears and nose closed it stays inside the body and activates the cells, gives new energy to each and every cell, tissue, organ, body and mind. It is a very simple pranayama with no side effect. Anyone can do it anywhere to de-stress and calm the busy mind.

Beneficial in - Tinnitus, vertigo, Cervical, Insomnia, sinus, migraine thyroid, relax nervous system, heart, boosts energy level, ADHD, autism, Height gain, hair fall, eyesight, seasonal allergies, anger

Not Recommended in – anyone can do it in moderation

How to do –

- Sit in comfortable position vajrasan, sukhasan keeping spine straight

- Focus on normal breathing (1 minute)

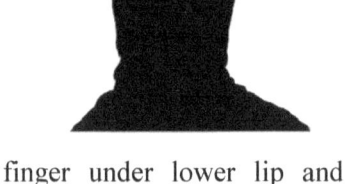

- Place index finger over the eyebrows, middle finger over eyes (press gently), ring finger partially closes nostrils, little finger under lower lip and thumb closing the ears from outside

- By covering our six senses (2 eyes, 2 ears, nose (partially closed) and mouth), we decrease the input of all the sensory inputs. It not only helps to focus and concentrate, it helps to keep the vibrations stay inside the body for longer period to gain the maximum benefit

- Inhale from nose

- Make hummm sound (like buzzing bee) while exhaling for as long as you can. Feel the vibrations inside the body for some time and then start with next round

- After every round, try to focus between eyebrows (agya chakra). If you feel discomfort gazing at Agya chakra then simply close eyes and feel the energy flow
- Repeat 5-7 times, end with exhalation and relax
- Once you are done, stay there in the position and feel the vibrations for about 2 minutes. Slowly open eyes and breathe normally

7) **Ujjayi (Ocean breath)** – 'Breath of Victory' or 'Ocean Breath' are other names for this pranayama. In the beginning, it may seem difficult but it's not. It brings more oxygen to the lungs, chest and brain which helps these organs to work better. It's a whispering sound which resembles like ocean waves by contracting vocal chords or glottis in the throat. It should be done to relax the body and mind.

Beneficial in – Thyroid, respiratory system, focus and concentration, improves quality of voice, re-energize body and mind, indigestion, to gain height, stuttering/stammering, snoring, insomnia, edema/dropsy

Not Recommended in – asthma, sciatica/ spinal injury, heart issues

How to do –
- Sit in comfortable posture vajrasan, sukhasan, padmasan with spine and neck straight
- Hands in gyan mudra on the knees
- Close eyes and focus on normal breath for 1 minute

- Put fingers of right hand on the throat to feel the air touching glottis
- Constrict throat and start inhaling from nose. The air isn't touching the nose walls rather they touch the throat wall and make a friction. This must sound like snoring
- Inhalation must be slow and long. Fill up lungs with as much air as you can. Your chest and then abdomen will expand. Hold the breath for 6 seconds
- Start exhaling firstly from abdomen, come up towards chest and then throat. Exhalation must also be slow and long with a sound like a ocean wave. Hold the breath
- Practice this for 3-5 minutes and then relax

Note* - During cold weather, one should never breathe through the mouth because the bronchial tubes become inflamed and congested

8) **Sheetali / Sheetkari** – These pranayama are useful to cool down body temperature. That's why they are recommended only during summers.

Beneficial in – reduces anger, fever, high BP, useful in mouth/tongue/throat diseases, indigestion, purifies blood, ADHD, depression, hyperactivity, insomnia

Not Recommended in – winters, low BP, asthma, cold and cough

How to do –
Sheetali pranayama

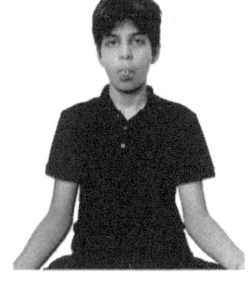

- Sit in a comfortable position vajrasan, sukhasan, padmasan
- Hands in gyan mudra on the knees
- Roll tongue and bring it forward between the lips
- Start inhaling from tongue as long as you can. When done hold the breath and close lips and lock the tongue inside and exhale slowly from nose
- Repeat for 3-5 minutes and relax

Sheetkari pranayama –

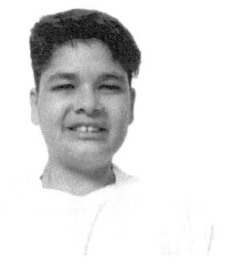

- Sit in meditative pose with hands in gyan mudra on knees
- Close eyes and roll tongue upward and touch the roof of the mouth
- Join upper and lower jaw and open lips
- Inhale/slurp the air with jaws closed. You will feel a cool breath inside the mouth. When done inhaling close lips and hold the breath for as long as you can and exhale from nose
- Repeat this for 3-5 minutes and relax

9) **Pranav pranayama (Om chanting)** – This can be said the first step to meditation. It allows you to focus on breath which helps to improve concentration level.

Beneficial in – High BP, insomnia, hypertension, migraine, during pregnancy, anger, anxiety, good practice to start meditation

Not recommended in – anyone can practice it

How to do –

- Sit in meditative pose with hands in gyan mudra
- Focus on normal breath for 2 minutes
- Inhale long and deep
- While exhaling, start chanting Om (with or without sound) bringing energy upward from tailbone flowing in spiral manner through spine and up towards crown chakra (top of the head)
- Breathe normally and this completes round one. After every round, feel the vibrations inside body with closed eyes
- Chant for 3-5 minutes and focus on normal breathing
- Rub your palms and place them on eyes and feel the warmth
- Start blinking eyes and see the light coming from fingers then slowly remove hands from eyes and relax

10) **Tratak (candle, moon, clock, god figure)** – It means to 'look' or to 'gaze' without blinking. This practice is also helpful in meditation especially for students and beginners. Gaze is fixed at one point during this meditation which helps an individual to focus more and increase concentration level.

Beneficial in – improves focus and concentration, eyesight, clears thoughts

Not Recommended in – glaucoma, after recent eye surgery

How to do –

- Find a secluded place (preferably dark room)

- Lit up a diya/candle and place it at a distance of 3-5 feet from your position (Diya is kept close in the image for clear view)

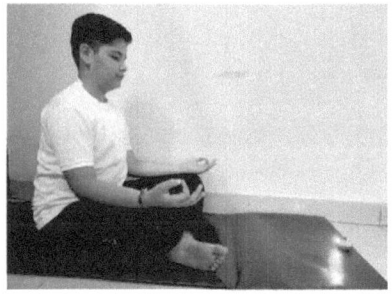

- Sit in meditative pose with hands in gyan mudra on knees

- Start gazing at the candle flame without blinking with complete focus on your breath

- Practice this for as long as you can. Close eyes, rub palms together and place them on the eyes. Feel the warmth and positive energy then start blinking and slowly see the light coming from the fingers and remove hands. Relax and breathe normally

Note* – You may gaze at moon, clock or God-figure as you like

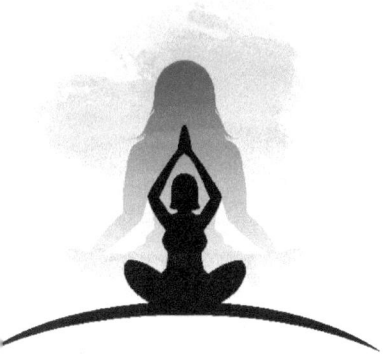

Chapter-7

Mudra

Hand Mudras are the hand gestures used in yog and dhyan to channelize the flow of energy in the body and brain. The five fingers represents five elements of which we are made of i.e, agni, vayu, akash, prithvi, jal (fire,air,space,earth,water). The energy activation point lies on the fingertips and when these point are connected the subtle energy in your body gets activated. They are applied in parallel with the meditation and asan. The mudras which are really useful during teenage years to combat emotional and physical hurricanes have been shared in this chapter.

Key points –

- All Mudras to be performed for about 10 min/day in the beginning then after a month of practice, increase it to 30-45 min/day

- Recommended to be practised in the morning and empty stomach

- Wear loose clothes for the free flow of energy
- Do not practice in 'extreme' stress, anger, anxiety like conditions
- Pregnant women must only practise asan, pranayama and mudra which are suggested 'Specifically for them' in the details.
- Restrict from smoking
- At any point of time if you start to feel uncomfortable, stop immediately.
- Do Not practice any specific mudra more than a month in continuity. Give a break for few days and then continue or do only till problem persists.

1) **Gyan mudra/Chin mudra** – This is the most used mudra in dhyan since ages. It helps to attain consciousness, knowledge and wisdom keeping your mind focused during meditation. It helps to sharpen memory, creativity, concentration and reduces impulsive thoughts. Since this is vayu vardhak mudra and increases vayu (air) element in the body.

Beneficial in - anger, anxiety, depression, insomnia, high bp, diabetes, heart disease and slows down Alzheimer

Not Recommended in – gas, acidity

How to do Gyan mudra–

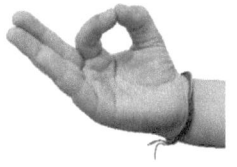

- Sit in comfortable position with spine and neck in one line.

- Keep your hands on your knees. Touch the tip of the index finger with tip of the thumb. Keep rest of the fingers in relaxed state facing upward.

- Practice this mudra while meditating. It helps to concentrate while keeping control on wandering thoughts.

- Do this mudra for 30-45 min/day or break it in 10min/3 times a day.

2) **Prana mudra** – This mudra improves the circulation of life force i.e, prana energy in the body which stimulates the nervous system, pituitary gland and chakras by supplying oxygen to nerves and cells of the body. It is also called kapha karak and pitta nashak mudra as three elements are working together- earth, water and fire which therefore, increases kapha dosh and eliminates pitta from the body. Hence, it is advised not to practise this mudra while having cold and cough.

Beneficial in – eye sight, high bp, diabetes, ulcers, aging skin, cramps, yawning, lethargy, weakness

Not Recommended in – runny nose, cold, cough, right after meal

How to do Prana mudra –

- Sit in comfortable position keeping spin and neck straight

- Touch the tip of ring and little finger to the tip of the thumb. Keep other fingers in relaxed state facing upwards.

- Practice this mudra for 30-45 min/day or break it in 10 min/3 times a day.

3) **Surya mudra –** As its name says it represents agni tatva (fire element) and hence, is also called agni vardhak mudra. It increases the heat in the body which helps in reducing cholesterol, improves digestion, metabolism, cures constipation which in turn helps in weight loss.

Beneficial in – weight loss, eye sight, coldness of hands and feet

Not Recommended in – underweight, fever, in summers, acidity, piles, ulcers, headache, acne, pregnancy, menstrual cycle

How to do Surya mudra –

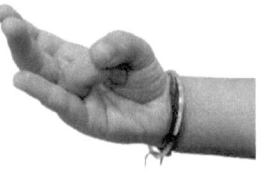

- Sit in comfortable position with spine and neck straight.

- Bend ring finger and touch the base of the thumb.

- Gently Press the finger with thumb. Keep rest of the fingers in relaxed state facing upwards.

- Practice this mudra for 30-45min/day after following do's and don'ts mentioned above and Only till problem persist.

4) **Yoni mudra** – It represents feminine energy (Shakti) and thus works for female reproductive organs, balances hormones which helps in keeping emotional stress at bay and helps to relieve physical pain and stomach cramps, provides fresh and rejuvenating energy to women during menstrual cycle. This mudra can be performed by men too to awaken the feminine energy (Shakti) with masculine energy (shiv) in the body to experience spiritual journey and overcome fertility problems.

Beneficial in – periods, pcos, menopause, emotional stress, infertility, pregnancy

Not Recommended in – high bp, extreme summers, fever, cold

How to do –

- Sit in comfortable position with spine and neck straight.
- Bend middle, ring and little fingers of both the hands. Make sure the back of the fingers of both the hands are touching each other facing upwards.
- Now join thumbs in upward direction and index finger downwards keeping them straight.
- Now position your hand in front of navel.

- Practice this mudra for 15-20 min/day after following dos and donts mentioned above and ONLY till problem persist.

5) **Ling mudra** – This mudra increases fire element in the body i.e, heat. It must be done in Winters or hypothermia like conditions to control body temperature. And can be performed only for 15-20 min/day. It can be practiced by both men and women as upright thumb represents masculine power and open palm represents feminine energy.

Note* - One should not practise this mudra for more than 15-20 min/day.

Beneficial in – regulating menstrual cycle, infections, wet cough, cold, shivering, sinusitis, asthma, bronchitis, weight loss (best when followed by surya mudra- both 15 min each), navel dislocation

Not Recommended in – high bp, acidity, fever, stomach ulcers

Note* - Do this mudra only till problem persists.

How to do –

- Sit in comfortable position with your spine and neck straight.
- There are two ways of doing ling mudra-
- First, interlock fingers and keep the right/left thumb in upright position, locking it with other thumb.

- Second, make a fist of right hand with thumb facing upward and place it on the left hand.

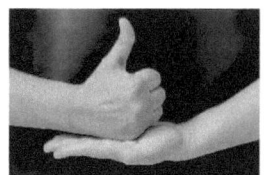

- Position this mudra in front of the navel

- Repeat this with other thumb facing upward.

6) **Hakini mudra** – Hakini is a Female Goddess, Energy, Power, diety of 6th chakra (Agya chakra). It gives you the power of intuition, clairvoyance, increases the coordination between both sides of the brain(left and right hemisphere). Thus, enhances concentration, thinking abilities. You must have seen many prominent people doing this mudra. Even when you want to concentrate more on something, you close your eyes and join your fingertips unintentionally and suddenly you are able to retrieve all the information you needed. Am I right? It really improves academic/ professional performance. Practice this for 30-45min/day.

Beneficial in – Clear thinking , enhances memory, improves concentration, improves brain functions, Autism, depression, dementia, alzhiemer, control blood pressure, pregnancy

Not Recommended in – injured wrist, weak physical and mental state

How to do –

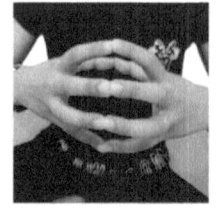

- Sit in comfortable position with spine straight.
- Join the tips of all fingers and thumb
- Position the hand in front of your chest

7) **Adi mudra** – Adi means first/primal. It is known as prime mudra/first gesture/ seal mudra. You must have noticed a baby inside and outside the womb makes this mudra in the initial days of his life which makes him feel calm and comfortable. It helps to calm down nervous system and stimulates brain cells which activates both left and right brain hemisphere, strengthens lungs capacity. Since, this mudra activates, energizes and balances the Sahasrar (Crown) Chakra, it enhances individuals higher awareness, sense of peace and oneness with the universe.

Beneficial in – balancing postures, lungs

Not Recommended in – wrist/thumb pain, during restlessness

How to do Adi mudra –

This mudra can be performed while sitting or standing.

- Keep your hands on your knees while sitting in meditative pose (sukhasan, padmaasan, vajrasan) with spine straight and eyes closed.

- While standing, do tadasan / stand straight maintaining distance between your hands and thighs.
- Touch the base of your little finger with your thumb and make a fist covering thumb with all fingers.
- Put gentle pressure on your thumb.
- Practice it for 45 min/day in continuity, else break it in three parts of 15min/ 3 times/ day

8) **Asthma mudra** – It relieves respiratory problems such as bronchitis, asthma, difficulty breathing. It activates the points of palms and fingers which corresponds to the lungs and chest. It creates warmth in the body which helps in clearing up nasal passage, chest congestion, removes phlegm, opens up bronchial tubes by supplying oxygen which in turn helps you to breathe properly.

Beneficial in- Bronchitis, Asthma, Allergies

Not Recommended in – weak wrist, weak physical state

How to do –

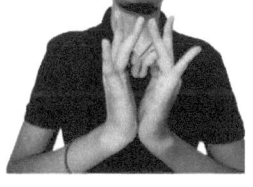

- Sit in comfortable position (sukhasan, padmasan, vajrasan) keeping spine and neck straight.
- Bring both of your hands in front of your chest facing each other.
- Fold middle fingers and touch their nails together.
- Now join end of your palms and try to keep rest of the fingers straight.

- Focus on breath
- Practice this for 10-15 min/day

NOTE – It may seem difficult to hold this mudra initially. Break 15 minutes into 5min/3 times/day.

9) **Varun mudra** – It is also called Water gesture/ Jal mudra. It balances water element in the body which helps in good blood circulation, kidney and liver function.

> As per my research, this mudra is helpful in overcome tinnitus problem as well. Here's a feedback - "Thank you so much for guiding me a mudra for my tinnitus problem. I am glad to share that my problem has been resolved in just 2 weeks. Much Gratitude! - Soni Kandhari, Dubai, UAE".

Beneficial in - anaemia, lowering cholesterol, urinary infections, improving low semen count, short menstruation cycle, gastroenteritis, skin glow

Not recommended in- cold and cough

How to do -

- Sit in a comfortable position with spine and neck in one line.

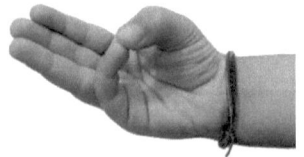

- Keep your hands on knees and touch the tip of the little finger with tip of the thumb. Keep rest of the fingers in relaxed state facing upwards.

- Practice it for 25-30 min/day or break it into 10 min/ 3 times a day.

10) **Shambhvi mudra** – This is an eye mudra and is practiced during the meditation. It is the powerful mudra to help stable the mind and experience higher stages of consciousness. You must have seen Adiyogi Shiv and many other great saints performing this mudra while sitting in dhyaan sadhna / Samadhi. It controls jnanaindreiya (sense organs) when you fix your gaze at one point i.e, agya chakra (point between eyebrows) which helps mind to settle down and hence random thoughts gets controlled.

Beneficial in – control sense organs, strengthen eye muscles, activates agya chakra, helps in meditation

Not recommended in – eye surgery, lens implant, glaucoma, migraine/vertigo (only do it under expert supervision)

How to do –

- Sit in comfortable position (sukhasan, padmasan, vajrasan). Hands in Gyan mudra on knees.

- Inhale and exhale with closed eyes – 2 rounds

- Open eyes while inhaling and focus your sight on the edge of the nose and exhale.

- Inhale and look up without moving head. Bring your sight to the centre of eyebrows (Agya chakra). You will notice eyebrows are joined together making a V shape.

- Chant OM while exhaling and keep looking at Agya chakra. Try to chant as long as possible.

- Close eyes and relax if you feel anxious, headache or dizzy and after 4-5 breaths you may start again.

11) **Shankh mudra** – Shankh means 'conch' and it is being held by Lord Vishnu which enhances courage, willpower, optimism and hope. It is very auspicious symbol and object of worship in indian culture. It's sound purifies the air and spreads positive vibes in the surroundings. Similarly, its mudra also has many benefits.

Beneficial in – sore throat, stammering, increase height, any kind of voice clarity specially after paralytic attack, balances thyroid hormones, allergies

Not Recommended in – wrist injury

How to do –

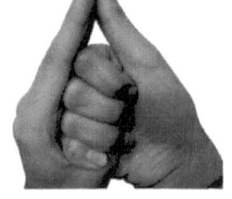

- Sit in sukhasan, padmasan, vajrasan

- Close/Open eyes and focus on breath

- Place your left thumb on right palm facing upward. Encircle it with right hand fingers and keep right thumb straight.

- Move left hand fingers facing upwards and touch middle finger to the right thumb, keeping other fingers straight.
- Place shankh mudra in front of the chest.
- Close eyes and chant OM in mind. You will start to hear the sound/vibrations within your body after sometime if practised properly.
- Do this mudra 10 min morning and evening.

12) **Bhramra mudra** – It means 'bee' in Sanskrit. The shape of hand resembles a bee. This mudra helps to get rid of all seasonal allergies like cold, skin rashes, itching etc.

Beneficial in – seasonal cold and allergies, asthma, bronchitis, runny/blocked/itchy nose, improves immune system

Not Recommended in – injured finger

How to do –
- Sit in sukhasan, vajrasan, padmasan
- Fold index finger and touch base of the thumb, touch tips of thumb and middle finger keeping other two fingers straight.
- Make this mudra in both hands. Place them in front of chest for about 10 minutes/3 times a day and focus on breath.

13) **Ganesh mudra** – It is named after Lord Ganesh hence it helps to overcome obstacles. With all fingers clasped together gives the power, energy, strength and a sense of security. It boosts metabolism as all panch tatva (5 elements) are bonded with each other. This mudra is performed in front of the chest/heart. It reduces the risk of heart diseases, improves function of lungs and digestion and strengthens muscle tissue. It helps to open heart chakra which stimulates love, compassion and feeling of inner joy.

Beneficial in – to relieve stress, worry, negative thoughts and depression

Not Recommended in – anyone can do it in moderation

How to do –

- Sit in comfortable position - sukhasan, padamasan

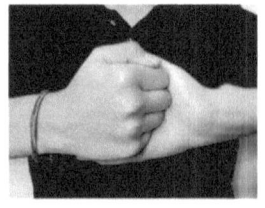

- Inhale, exhale and relax your breath and body

- Make anjali mudra (namaskar mudra) in front of the chest

- Now turn hands in horizontal position opposite to each other. Right hand fingers touch base of left palm and left hand fingers touch base of right palm.

- Make a clasp with fingers

- Cover the fist with right thumb from above and left thumb from below

- The interlock fist is energetically pulled apart without releasing the grip in front of the chest
- Stay in this posture for atleast 10 min during meditation
- Change the side of the hand and repeat
- Invoke the Lord and its power by chanting his name in the form of mantra 'Om Ganpataye Namah'

14) **Prithvi mudra** – Prithvi means Earth. In this mudra when earth element meets fire element, it gives the power of stability, builds confidence and bodily strength, get rid of confusion, anxiety, fearfulness, fickle mindedness. It is also helpful in gaining weight and hair growth.

Recommended in – weight gain, physical weakness, indecisiveness

Not Recommended in – asthma, overweight, cough

How to do –

- Sit in sukhasan, padmasan with spine and neck straight

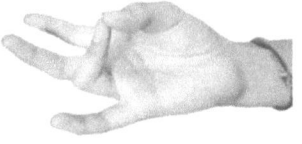

- Breathe and relax yourself. Place hands on knees
- Touch the ring finger tip to the tip of the thumb. Do this with both the hands simultaneously
- Let the rest of the fingers be straight facing upward in relaxed manner

- Breathe and stay in the position for about 30-45 min in one go or 10 min/3 times a day

15) **Apan mudra** – This mudra channelizes the flow of energy towards lower abdominal region which helps in digestive and excretory problems.

Beneficial in – constipation, indigestion, acidity, urinary problems, eases childbirth, menstrual cramps, body detoxification, toothache

Not Recommended in – during first 8 months of pregnancy, diarrhea, dysentery, cholera

How to do –
- Sit in sukhasan, padmasan, vajrasan and keep spine straight

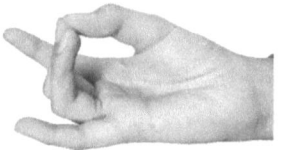

- Relax your breath and body. Keep both hands on knees

- Touch the tip of thumb with tip of ring and middle finger. Keep index and little finger relaxed. Do this with both the hands simultaneously.

- Focus on your breath and visualise the energy flowing towards you pelvic region/lower abdominal region

- Stay in the position for 30-45 min/day or 10 min/3 times a day

Note* - Apan mudra is not suggested in first 8 months of pregnancy. If done, one may face miscarriage. And if done during childbirth, it eases the labour pain.

16) **Vayu mudra** – This mudra regulates the air element in the body. It helps in alleviating different pains in the body like rheumatic arthritis, joint pains, sciatica, gastric disorders and psychological disorders like Parkinson disease symptoms, stimulates endocrine glands to secret hormones for proper growth. It helps brain to function properly by providing oxygen.

Beneficial in – arthritis, gas, forgetfulness, balance hormones

Not Recommended in- anyone can do it in moderation

How to do –

- You may do this mudra while sitting, standing or walking

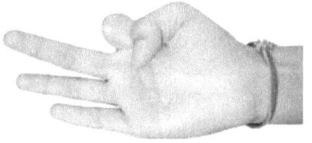

- Bend index finger and touch the base of the thumb. Put gentle pressure on the finger
- Keep rest of the three fingers straight
- Do this mudra for 30-45 min or 10 min/ 3 times a day

17) **Apanvayu mudra** – This is the mudra for heart as it reduces the effect of heart attack, palpitations by balancing all three dosh(vata, kapha, pitt). It controls vata (air) and balances apan energy which cleanses the intestines and eases gastric issues.

Beneficial in- heart related problems, artery blockage, palpitations, high bp, anxiety, nervousness, improves lung capacity and digestion

Not recommended in – pregnancy (only under supervision)

How to do –

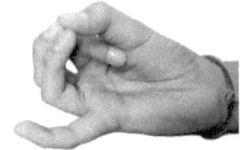

- You may sit/stand/ lie down keeping spine straight
- Place hands on knees, close eyes and relax your breath
- Fold index finger and touch the base of the thumb
- Touch the tip of the thumb with tips of middle and ring finger. keep little finger straight but in relaxed manner
- Do this with each hand simultaneously for 30-45 min

18) **Bhrama mudra** – This mudra is named after lord Bhrama, the creator of the Universe, who has four heads. This mudra has two parts- hast mudra and neck rotation which is done while chanting Om mantra.

Beneficial in – releases negative energy and thoughts, detoxification, releases pain stiffness in neck shoulders and upper back, stimulates digestive system, nervous system and respiratory system

Not recommended in – cold, cough, fever

How to do –

- Sit in sukhasan, padmasan, vajrasan

- Place both hands in front of navel, palms facing upwards

- Touch the base of little finger with respective thumb

- Wrap thumb with all fingers over and around and make a fist

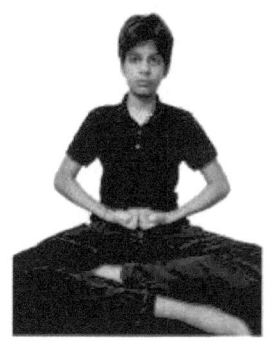

- Join and press the knuckles of both fists as shown in the pic

- Do this for 30-45 min or 15 min twice a day

How to do Bhrama mudra neck rotation –

- Sit straight, inhale and focus at one point in front you

- Start to chant Om in your mind

- Exhale and look up. Stretch throat completely and fix your gaze at nose tip

- Inhale come back to centre

- Exhale, bend your head down and touch chin with collarbone

- Inhale come back to centre

- Exhale, turn head towards right side and look back as far as possible

- Inhale come back to centre

- Exhale, turn head towards left side and look back as far as possible

- Inhale come back to centre

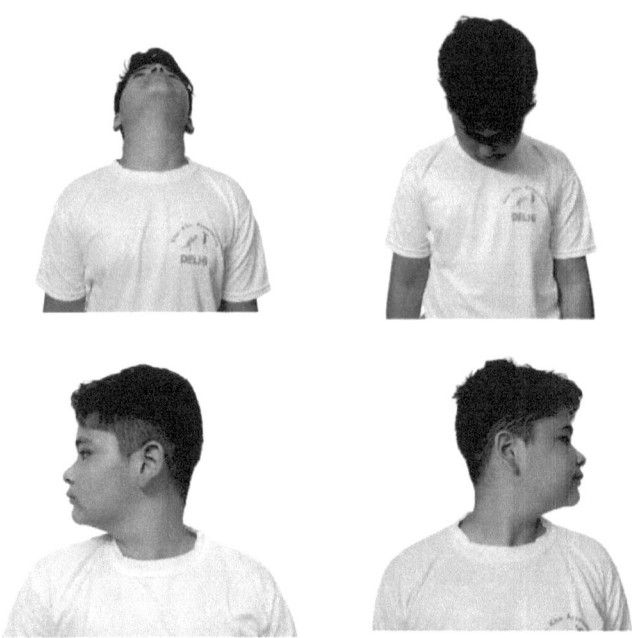

Note*- Maintain breath-work as suggested during all movements

19) **Vajra mudra** – It is a powerful mudra to get rid of laziness and feel energetic quickly. 'Vajra' means weapon and it is the weapon of God Indra. By performing this mudra consistently, blood circulation gets better in the spinal cord and clears the toxins, blockages from the blood and helps to

activate chakras. It also helps in getting rid of toxic traits of the person.

Beneficial in – Circulatory system, helps in quitting smoke/ drink habits, cuts down on tea/ caffeine, regain energy, detoxify lungs, purifies blood, sharpens brain, increases memory

Not recommended in – high BP patients

How to do –

- Sit in a comfortable position in sukhasan, vajrasan, padmasan keeping spine and neck straight

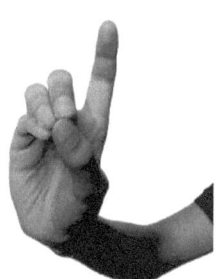

- Both hands on knees with palms facing up. Close eyes

- Fold middle, ring and little fingers and gently press the tip of the thumb while index fingers remains straight pointing forward.

- Do this with both the hands together and focus on breath

- Now, fold the tongue back in mouth and touch the tip to the top of the mouth (palate)

- Practice this for 20 minutes/ a day or 7 minutes/ 3 times a day

Note* – high BP patients can do for 5 minutes maximum under supervision

20) **Merudand mudra** – This is called spine mudra as 'meru' means spine. It helps to heal, reenergise and

activate spinal cord. This helps circulation of breath in lower back and hips and enhances Manipur chakra which increases confidence, determination and balances cluttered mind.

Beneficial in – strengthens spine, weight loss in thighs and hips, improves determination and confidence, detox liver and spine

Not Recommended in – High BP (under supervision)

How to do –

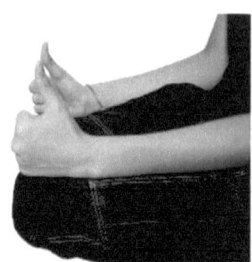

- Sit comfortably in any position keeping spine and neck straight

- Make a loose fists with thumbs pointing up

- Place hands on thighs and start to focus on breath

- Stay in the position for 5-10 minutes

21) **Shunya mudra** – Shunya literally means nothing. In yog, it refers to emptiness as it reduces space element in the body.

Beneficial in – hearing loss, tinnitus, improves balance, manage dizziness, vertigo

Not Recommended in – recent undergone ear surgery

How to do –

- You can do this mudra while sitting / standing / walking

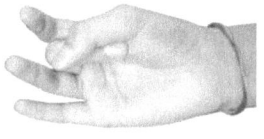

- Fold and touch the tip of the middle finger to the base of the thumb

- Cover the middle finger with thumb

- Keep rest of the fingers straight in relaxed manner

- Focus on breath

- Hold this mudra for 30 minutes a day or 10 minutes 3 times a day

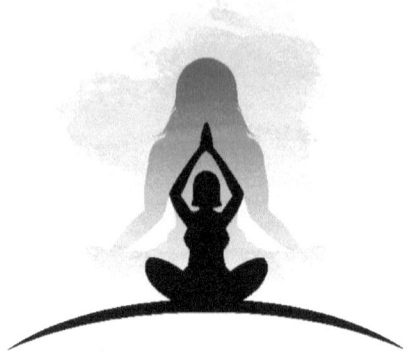

Chapter-8

Meditation

There are different kinds of meditations which are practised all over the world. Every school teaches their own kind of relaxation technique. Its main purpose is to relax body and calm the mind while making a connection between body, breath and mind. It's best when practised after yogasan and pranayama as the body's nervous system is active and breath is fully under control.

Practising Mindfulness meditations makes you live in present moment, helps you to accept everything as is, keeps you happy and stress free of past and future worries.

Types of Dhyan–

- Chakra healing and balancing
- Spiritual meditation

- Transcendental meditation – silently repeat mantra in mind
- Mantra meditation – chant mantra loudly or quietly
- Antaryatra (Internal Trip)
- Dharna (Focused meditation) focus on internal or external influences like breath, candle flame, counting mala beads, gazing at moon/God pic)
- Preksha Dhyan (Visualization meditation/ body scan)
- Anupreksha (Contemplation)
- Kayotsarg (Relaxation technique)

Amongst all, only one technique is being explained here to make it easier for you to understand to start with and practice as a beginner.

Spiritual Meditation – Connect with the Universe

Spirituality isn't related to any religion. It simply means 'Connect with the Supreme Power' and Meditation is a tool that helps you achieve it.

There are different variations for all types of practitioners. Start with your own suitability -

- Lie down on the mat with arms on the side of your body, feet half feet apart (for beginners)

    or

- Sit straight with spine and neck in one line. Hands in Gyan mudra (check Mudras) resting on knees or

Vitrag mudra (place right hand flat over left hand) close to navel (for intermediate practitioners)

or

- Stand straight with arms on the side, legs half feet apart, eyes closed. This is the most difficult posture to meditate. It is not recommended for beginners as they may fall asleep and injure themselves (for experts only)

As your breath is calm and steady after pranayama, close your eyes and take two long and deep breaths. Start to look at the centre of the eyebrows (agna chakra) and keep on breathing normally. You will see your muscles are getting loosened up and body is falling down (relaxed) after every breath and keep looking at the centre of the eyebrow. After sometime, you will be able to control your thoughts on your own. And that comes with regular practice.

After you choose the posture, gently close your eyes and start to breathe. Pay attention to every breath you take in and giving out. Inhale positivity, love, peace, joy, happiness and Exhale all the negativity, hatred, anger, fear, guilt and toxins from your body. Relax with every breath. Now focus on third eye/ agya chakra/ centre of consciousness located between eyebrows. You will only see dark, hollow space. Keep looking at it for sometime with relaxed breathing. Your mind will definitely be wandering, let it be and come back to focus on your breathing. Now its time to connect with the universe. In your thoughts, convey the message to the universe 'I need universal energy to heal my body, mind and soul'.

Repeat this 3 times and wait. After a while, visualise a bright ray of light coming from the universal space. Its beautiful pure white light and it's coming towards you, entering your body from the top of your head / crown chakra. The white particles of the light are spreaded in your head. Universal energy works really fast. It can heal and repair in no time. White light particles are reaching to every tissue, neuron, cell in your brain giving them new energy, new life. Neurons are getting charged, tissues are getting repaired, cells are re-energising. Each and every part of the brain is receiving this healing energy. Inhale and exhale. Feel the happiness within and let release happy hormones in your body, you may feel a little shiver/goosebumps while doing so. Relax, inhale and exhale. Your mind is at complete relaxed state and so is your body. Slowly, come back to consciousness and try to move your fingers. Join your hands to do namaskar mudra/ Anjali mudra. Pay heartfelt gratitude to the universe for providing this powerful healing energy, for prana energy which keeps us alive, for this precious life, for beautiful family and friends, for everything we have. Now pay gratitude to the Mother Earth for feeding us and nourishing us. In the end, Rub your palms together and feel the heat energy in your hands and place them on your face with a thought that you are locking this supreme healing energy in your body and then take your hands towards head, neck, shoulders, arms, chest, abdomen, mid-back, lower back, thighs, calves and feet. Again, rub your palms and place them on your eyes, start blinking and slowly open eyes in the darkness of your hands, let the light come in from the fingers and see the light. Remove hands from the face and smile. I welcome you back and thank you for taking the session. Hope you enjoyed every moment of it and feel completely relaxed with a fresh energy in mind and body.

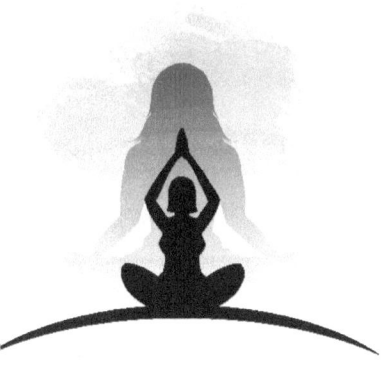

CHAPTER-9

Shuddhi Kriya - Cleansing techniques

1) Kapalbhati
2) Nasya basti (oil, ghee)
3) Netra shuddhi (oil, ghee, triphala, water)

1) **Kapalbhati** - It is also called 'skull shining'. It removes toxins, excess carbon dioxide from the body, strengthens core and chest, and energises circulatory, respiratory and nervous system.

Note*:

i) A beginner must practise basic breathing techniques before trying kapalbhati.

ii) Patients of High BP, ulcers, heart and respiratory problems, slip disc must practice only under expert supervision

iii) Women during pregnancy and periods should not practice it.

iv) Kapalbhati must be practised in the beginning of the session before asan and pranayama.

How to do Kapalbhati -

1) Sit comfortably in sukhasan, padmasan or vajrasan with spine and neck straight.

2) Place hands in gyan mudra on knees

3) Take a long and deep breath and fill the abdomen with air. (You may place left hand on the navel if you are a beginner to feel the exhalations)

4) Now start forceful exhalations without active inhalations.

5) While exhaling, pull your navel button as close to the spine (feel contraction and relaxation of abdominal muscles)

6) Start with 15-20 exhalations in one go and do 5 rounds i.e, about 100 exhalations. Slowly increase the number over a period of time and try to exhale 100 times in one go and do 3 rounds i.e, 300 times in total.

7) You may take a break after every round (i.e, after 20 breaths) and breathe normally 3 times and repeat the process.

8) In the end, close eyes and feel the vibrations happening in your body and brain. The energy is moving and clearing up all the toxins from the body. This is the time you get connected with your breath, body, mind and soul. Enjoy the moment!

2) Nasya basti (oil, ghee)

Nasya basti (Nasal cleansing process) – It is a simple procedure to cleanse and detox nasal passage. It is an ayurvedic treatment which has been followed by our parents inherited by our ancestors, rishi and sages from thousands of years. Oiling or lubricating nasal passage has multiple benefits. It can be done once/twice a day with sesame oil/ mustard oil/ desi ghee (clarified butter). Preferred period is winters as skin is dry and rough, nasal passage is blocked with mucus. This is suitable for people aged between 7-80 years.

Beneficial in – Helpful in Sinus, cold/flu, throat, migraine, headache, eyesight, hairfall, seasonal allergies, skin glow

Not Recommended in – acute fever, just before/after shower

How to do –

Half hour Before/After shower, take little amount of oil/ghee on finger, close one nostril and inhale from another and repeat from other nostril. Make sure the oil reaches the throat via nostrils.

✓ A quick tip –

- Rub a little amount of desi ghee on hands, feet and face in winters to get the glow
- Rub some ghee on chest and throat in the night to get rid of mucus, cough, cold and flu

3) **Netra shuddhi(oil, ghee, triphala, water)**

   Netra shuddhi (eye wash)- This procedure might look difficult to some but it's not. Washing eyes properly gives the soothing effect to the optic nerves, removes burning and tiredness of eyes which helps in improving eye sight if done regularly. Effect can only be seen after practising for atleast 4-5 months.

Beneficial in – improving eyesight, removes burning and puffiness of eyes, soothes watery or sore eyes, dark circles, overcome insomnia

Not Recommended in – any eye injury or undergone eye surgery recently

How to do –

Eye wash can be done with oil, ghee, triphala powder or water. For beginners, water is recommended to start with. You will need a pair of eye wash cups (which is available online). Sanitize them with lukewarm water and a little salt before using them for the first time.

- Fill eye wash cups with clean water

- Add a pinch of rock salt (optional)

- Bend down your head and place the cups onto the eyes. When cups make a vaccum and stick to the eyes, look up

- Keep eyes opened and start to rotate the eyeballs clockwise and then anti-clockwise direction

- Start blinking eyes rapidly

- To release, bend down again and slowly remove the cups
- Repeat it 2-3 times a day

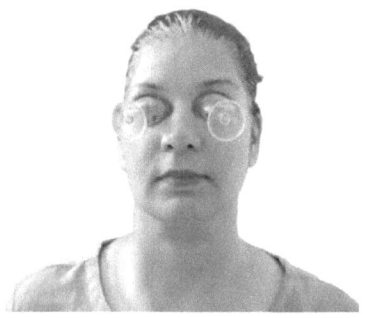

Note* – Eye wash cups are specific for each person in the house just like a toothbrush and cannot be used by everyone in the family. To use oil, ghee or triphala powder- expert supervision is needed.

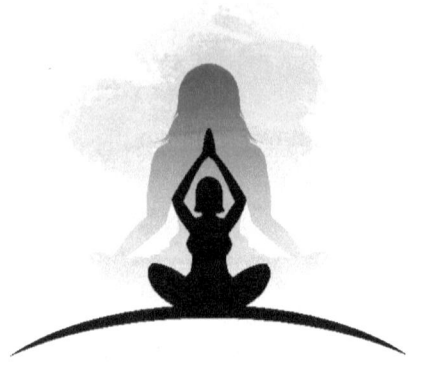

Chapter-10

Solution to Physical, Mental and Social Issues

S.no.	Issue	Yogasan	Pranayam	Mudra/shudhi kriya
1.	Obesity	Surya namaskar, katichakarasan, trikonasan, mandukasan, vipritkarni asan	bhastrika, anulom-vilom	Surya mudra, ling mudra, kapalbhati
2.	Eyesight	suksham vyayam (eyes), adhomukhsavasan, halasan, sarvangasan, ushtrasan, padhastasan	Tratak, bhastrika, bhramri	Shambhavi mudra, Prana mudra, surya mudra, netra shuddh, nasya basti
3.	Height	Tadasan, vrikshasan, parvatasan, chakrasan, bhujangasan, sarvangasan, ushtrasan	Ujjayi, pranav pranayama (om chanting), bhramri	Prana mudra, shankh mudra

4.	Acne, Hairfall	Viprit karni, sarvangasan, halasan, uttanasan, matsyasan, ushtrasan, adhomukhsvanasan, shirshasan	Anulom-vilom,	Prithvi mudra, prana mudra, kapalbhati
5.	Learning disorder – ADHD	Surya namaskar, Balasan, mandukasan, vipritkarni, trikonasan, badhkonasan, savasan	Bhramri, Om chanting, sheetali, sheetkari, rhythmic breathing	Gyan mudra, hakini mudra
6.	Asthma /Bronchitis/Lung Cancer	Gomukhasa, bhujangasan, ushtrasan, simhasan	Bhastrika, anulom-vilom	Asthma mudra, ling mudra, kapalbhati,
7.	Autism spectrum disorder (Asd)/ Autism	Vrikshasan, virbhadrasan, utakatkonasan(Goddess pose), badhkonasan, savasan	Bhramri, Om chanting, rhythmic breathing	Ganesh mudra, hakini mudra
8.	Chronic Fatique syndrome (Cfs)	vrikshasan, trikonasan, balasan, bhujangasan, vajrasan, suptbadhkonasan, savasan	Bhastrika, anulom vilom, Rhythmic breathing	Prana mudra, Gyan mudra, ling mudra, ganesh mudra
9.	Hearing (Tinnitus, vertigo)	subtle exercise(Ear), sarvang asan, halasan, adhomukhsavasan	Bhramri	Shunya mudra
10.	Digestive issues - Ulcers, IBS, GERD Hernia	Vajrasan, marjaryasan-bitilasan, bhujangasan, suptbadhkonasan	rhythmic breathing, anulom-vilom	Apan mudra, vayu mudra

11.	Constipation, Indigestion	uttanasan, vajrasan, marjaryasan-bitilasan, kati-chakrasan	Deergh (Deep breathing)	Apanvayu mudra, kapalbhati
12.	Cold and flu	Vipritkarni, halasan, chakrasan, uttanasan, ear massage (subtle exercise)	Suryabhedna, deergh (deep breathing), anulom-vilom	Surya mudra, ling mudra
13.	Psoriasis	Practice all asan regularly	All pranayams are beneficial	Varun mudra, apply (curd) or (buttermilk) or (turmeric, garlic oil, aloevera) on the affected area.
14.	Blood disorder– Anaemia Diabetes Thalassemia	Trikonasan, balasan, adhomukhsvasan, Parvatasan, sarvangasan	Bhastrika, anulom-vilom	Vajra mudra, prithvi mudra, prana mudra
15.	Tennis elbow	Gomukhasan, shalabhasan with arms under the body palms facing downwards	All pranayama are beneficial	Prana mudra
16.	Cervical	Makarasan, Gomukhasan, bhujangasan, Merudandasa, neck exercises	Suryabhedn, bhramri	Ling mudra, merudand mudra, kapalbhati

17.	Sinus/ Migraine/ Hairfall/ Seasonal allergies	Matsyasan, ustrasan, adhomukhsvasan, sarvangasan, Parvatasan	Anulom-vilom, bhramri	Ling mudra, gyan mudra, shankh mudra, bhramra mudra, Nasya basti, kapalbhati
18.	Speech disorders/ stuttering	Matsyasan, simhasan, bhujangasan, mouth exercises	Ujjayi, bhastrika, bhramri,	Brahma mudra, shankh mudra, kapalbhati
19.	Depression/ Anxiety	Surya Namaskar, Uttan shishosana (puppy pose), uttanasan, balasan, savasan	Sheetali, sheetkari, anulom-vilom, Om chanting	Apan vayu mudra, gyan mudra, hakini mudra, kapalbhati
20.	Anger	Surya namaskar, simhasan, chakrasan, Uttan shishosana (puppy pose), ardh pinch mayurasan (dolphin pose), balasan, sarvangasan, savasan	Sheetali, sheetkari, bhramri	Hakini mudra, shankh mudra, gyan mudra

Note:

1) The above mentioned illnesses/disorders can be avoided, delayed or improve the condition to a great extent with the help of yoga. Yoga isn't the cure but a preventive measure.

2) Meditation is must for all and to be practised in the end.

3) There are more asan, pranayama and mudras which are beneficial but the few mentioned above are specifically for each illness and will give maximum benefit.

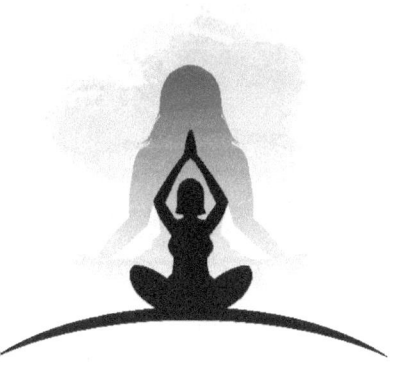

Chapter-11

FAQ's- Frequently asked Questions

Q 1. Is yoga safe for Children? At what age should a child start yoga?

Yes, Children can start practising asan from the age of 5 and shuddhi kriya (Cleansing technique) from 12 yrs and above under expert supervision.

Q 2. How do you explain yoga to a child?

Yoga can be fun activity for children. We can explain the animal postures and its benefits like how it helps to gain bodily strength like a lion, flexibility like a cobra, add laughter yoga which boosts up mood.

Q 3. How do I teach my 5 year old to be stable and focused?

Handling a 5 year old is not easy and we cannot expect him to sit stable and be focussed. We need to engage him/her in conversation while performing asan by telling/sharing stories or making sounds of the animal which is being practised at that moment. Tratak meditation will help him get better with regular practice.

Q 4. How do I explain a child that yoga is better than mobile phone?

Mobile phone has taken an edge off everything. Yes, I agree that it's difficult to take away phones and indulge them in other activity. But a parent can do anything. Limit the phone time and make a time table and encourage child to follow the routine by encouraging and motivating him for small tasks completed. Now add yoga in timetable and start with 20 min daily practice. Gradually, add pranayam and meditation and see the difference in your child.

Q 5. Do I need to practice with him/her?

Initially yes, if you want your child to continue this routine. Moreover, doing yoga with you will motivate him.

Q 6. Is meditation good for my child?

Yes, meditation has many benefits for all age groups.

Q 7. Can a child with physical / mental disabilities perform yoga? Is it safe for them?

Yoga is safe for everyone if practised under expert supervision.

Q 8. Can a child admitted in hospital do yoga?

Yes, definitely. Pranayama and meditation can be done properly but only limited asan can be performed with limited movements. Recovery is seen in many patients who practiced yoga in hospital.

Q 9. Can yoga remove spectacles ?

It takes time but yes. Regular practice of asan, eye exercises, netra shuddhi, pranayama has proven to improve the eyesight and remove spectacles.

Q 10. Can yoga improve my child in studies ?

Yoga improves focus and concentration which helps a child to learn and comprehend easily which results in good academic performance.

Q 11. Does yoga help in increasing height ?

Yogasan are full of stretching muscles and lengthening spine like tadasan, vrikshasan, parvatasan, adhomukh savasan etc. Inverted postures helps to stimulate pineal gland which helps in gaining height. Meditation relaxes and calms the mind, which helps to produce growth hormones during teenage years.

Review

"Yoga for Next Generation "by Gayatri is more than just a yoga manual; it is a compassionate guide that addresses the multifaceted lives of teenagers. By combining physical postures with mindfulness practices, Bhaskar provides teens with valuable tools to navigate their formative years with greater ease and confidence. This book is a must-read for children, parents, and educators alike, offering a pathway to holistic health and well-being.

As a yogaguru, I highly recommend this book for its thoughtful integration of yoga and mindfulness, and its ability to meet teens where they are, both physically and emotionally.

Best wishes

Yogaguru Shailendra

Founder: The Yogaguru Institute

Pre and post-natal Yoga expert

A Note of Thanks

First and foremost, I would like to pay my gratitude to the Almighty who has always been kind to me. Universe has blessed me in every possible way by showing the right path.

I am obliged to my parents for bringing me into this beautiful world and teaching me good values in my childhood, which helped me to get into yoga and spirituality at an early age and living a blissful life.

I wholeheartedly express my thanks to G. Rajaraman, who has inspired and motivated me to write. He is the driving force behind this book.

I, now acknowledge Gagan Adhlakha, my mentors - Shailendra sir and Mohan sir for their valuable reviews about the book.

My family has always been a big support in all my ventures. My husband Kapil, who is my backbone and the first one to push me to do what I like. My son Karan, a teenager who always understands me and my work. They always showed their faith in me and have been a great help till now. Their support makes a huge difference in my life. After becoming a mother, I never felt a setback. And ofcourse, my fur baby-Kookie for her understanding and waiting for her playtime while I work. Thank you all for your unconditional love.

I would also like to express my gratitude to my students and their parents who took time for the photo shoot and showed their skills to the utmost level. A big hug to all - Jaisvi, Aadiv, Vanya, Khayati, Karan, Shaurya and Anant.

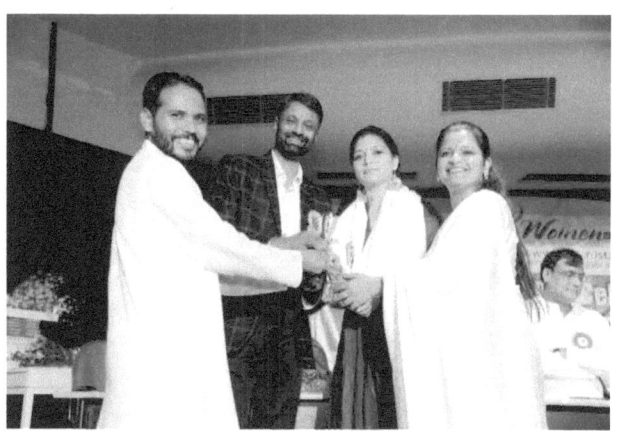

Honoured by Yogagurus

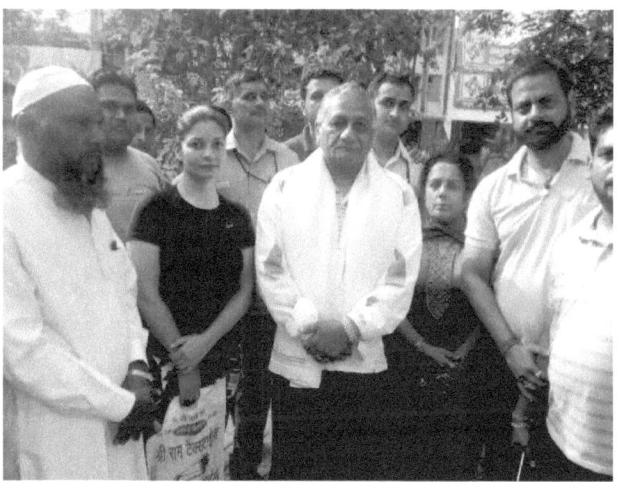

Honoured by V.K.Singh, MP Loksabha

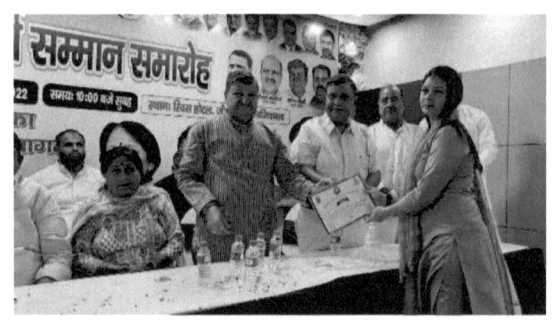

Achievers Award 2022 by MP Sh. Anil Aggarwal and MLA Sh. Atul Garg

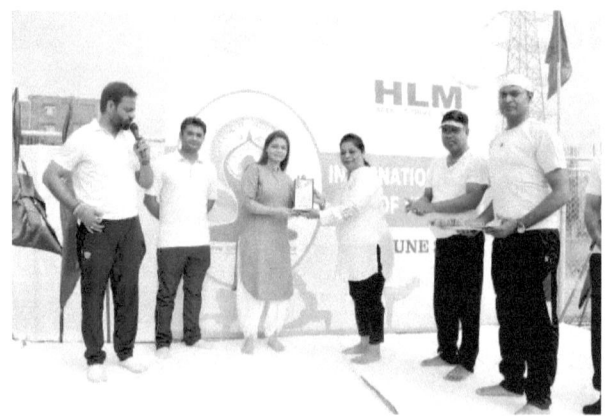

Honoured by HLM group on International Yoga day'22

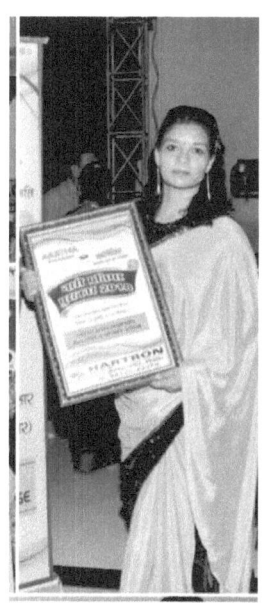
Women Achievers Award

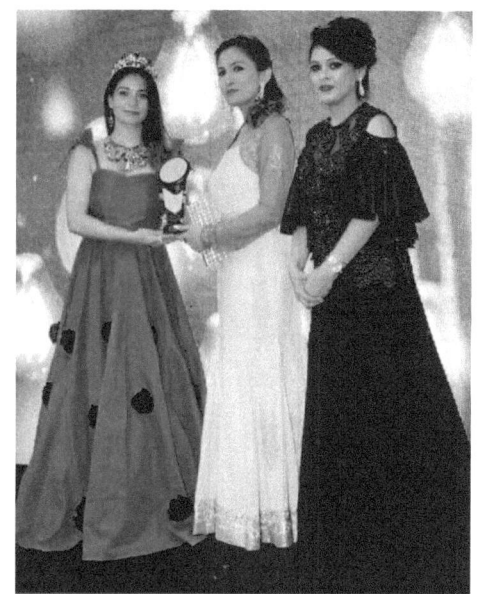
Guest of honour -Mrs India 2017

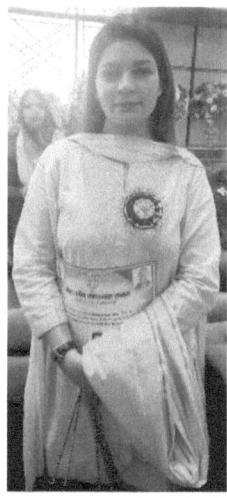
Mahila Shakti Jagrukta Samman'23

www.ingramcontent.com/pod-product-compliance
Lightning Source LLC
LaVergne TN
LVHW041849070526
838199LV00045BA/1508